35

Reproductive Genetics

Editor

LORRAINE DUGOFF

OBSTETRICS AND GYNECOLOGY CLINICS OF NORTH AMERICA

www.obgyn.theclinics.com

Consulting Editor
WILLIAM F. RAYBURN

March 2018 • Volume 45 • Number 1

ELSEVIER

1600 John F. Kennedy Boulevard • Suite 1800 • Philadelphia, Pennsylvania, 19103-2899

http://www.theclinics.com

OBSTETRICS AND GYNECOLOGY CLINICS OF NORTH AMERICA Volume 45, Number 1
March 2018 ISSN 0889-8545, ISBN-13: 978-0-323-58164-6

Editor: Kerry Holland
Developmental Editor: Kristen Helm

Obstetrics and Gynecology Clinics (ISSN 0889-8545) is published quarterly by Elsevier Inc., 360 Park Avenue South, New York, NY 10010-1710. Months of issue are March, June, September, and December. Periodicals postage paid at New York, NY, and additional mailing offices. Subscription price per year is $313.00 (US individuals), $652.00 (US institutions), $100.00 (US students), $393.00 (Canadian individuals), $823.00 (Canadian institutions), $225.00 (Canadian students), $459.00 (international individuals), $823.00 (international institutions), and $225.00 (international students). To receive student/resident rate, orders must be accompanied by name of affiliated institution, date of term, and the signature of program/residency coordinator on institution letterhead. Orders will be billed at individual rate until proof of status is received. Foreign air speed delivery is included in all *Clinics* subscription prices. All prices are subject to change without notice. POSTMASTER: Send address changes to *Obstetrics and Gynecology Clinics*, Elsevier Health Sciences Division, Subscription Customer Service, 3251 Riverport Lane, Maryland Heights, MO 63043. **Customer Service: Telephone: 1-800-654-2452 (U.S. and Canada); 314-447-8871 (outside U.S. and Canada). Fax: 314-447-8029. E-mail: journalscustomerservice-usa@elsevier.com (for print support); journalsonlinesupport-usa@elsevier. com (for online support).**

Reprints. For copies of 100 or more of articles in this publication, please contact the Commercial Reprints Department, Elsevier Inc., 360 Park Avenue South, New York, New York 10010-1710. Tel.: 212-633-3874; Fax: 212-633-3820; E-mail: reprints@elsevier.com.

Obstetrics and Gynecology Clinics of North America is also published in Spanish by McGraw-Hill Interamericana Editores S.A., P.O. Box 5-237, 06500, Mexico; in Portuguese by Reichmann and Affonso Editores, Rio de Janeiro, Brazil; and in Greek by Paschalidis Medical Publications, Athens, Greece.

Obstetrics and Gynecology Clinics of North America is covered in MEDLINE/PubMed (Index Medicus), Excerpta Medica, Current Concepts/Clinical Medicine, Science Citation Index, BIOSIS, CINAHL, and ISI/BIOMED.

Contributors

CONSULTING EDITOR

WILLIAM F. RAYBURN, MD, MBA
Associate Dean, Continuing Medical Education and Professional Development, Distinguished Professor and Emeritus Chair, Obstetrics and Gynecology, The University of New Mexico School of Medicine, Albuquerque, New Mexico

EDITOR

LORRAINE DUGOFF, MD
Professor, Obstetrics and Gynecology, Director, Reproductive Genetics, Divisions of Maternal Fetal Medicine and Reproductive Genetics, University of Pennsylvania Perelman School of Medicine, Philadelphia, Pennsylvania

AUTHORS

MEGAN A. ALLYSE, PhD
Center for Bioethics, Mayo Clinic, Rochester, Minnesota

WHITNEY BENDER, MD
Department of Obstetrics and Gynecology, Hospital of the University of Pennsylvania, Philadelphia, Pennsylvania

ANUJA DOKRAS, MD, PhD
Professor of Obstetrics and Gynecology, Division of Reproductive Endocrinology and Infertility, Department of Obstetrics and Gynecology, University of Pennsylvania, Philadelphia, Pennsylvania

LORRAINE DUGOFF, MD
Professor, Obstetrics and Gynecology, Director, Reproductive Genetics, Divisions of Maternal Fetal Medicine and Reproductive Genetics, University of Pennsylvania Perelman School of Medicine, Philadelphia, Pennsylvania

RUTH M. FARRELL, MD, MA
OB/GYN and Women's Health Institute, Department of Bioethics, Cleveland Clinic, Cleveland, Ohio

KRISTIN D. GERSON, MD, PhD
Department of Obstetrics and Gynecology, Beth Israel Deaconess Medical Center, Department of Obstetrics, Gynecology, and Reproductive Biology, Harvard Medical School, Boston, Massachusetts

ANTHONY R. GREGG, MD, MBA
Professor, Chief Maternal Fetal Medicine, Department of Obstetrics and Gynecology, University of Florida College of Medicine, Gainesville, Florida

JENNIFER M. HOSKOVEC, MS, CGC
Department of Obstetrics, Gynecology and Reproductive Sciences, McGovern Medical School, The University of Texas Health Science Center at Houston, Houston, Texas

ANGIE C. JELIN, MD
Division of Maternal-Fetal Medicine, Department of Gynecology and Obstetrics, The Johns Hopkins University School of Medicine, Baltimore, Maryland

DANIEL KASER, MD
Reproductive Medicine Associates of New Jersey, Basking Ridge, New Jersey

JENNIFER R. KING, MD, MS, FACOG
Department of Obstetrics and Gynecology and Women's Health, Division of Reproductive and Medical Genetics, Albert Einstein College of Medicine, Montefiore Medical Center, Bronx, New York

SUSAN KLUGMAN, MD, FACOG, FACMG
Department of Obstetrics and Gynecology and Women's Health, Division of Reproductive and Medical Genetics, Albert Einstein College of Medicine, Montefiore Medical Center, Bronx, New York

BRYNN LEVY, MSc (Med), PhD
Professor, Department of Pathology and Cell Biology, Columbia University Medical Center, New York, New York

SUSAN C. MODESITT, MD, FACOG, FACS
Professor and Director, Division of Gynecologic Oncology, Department of Obstetrics and Gynecology, University of Virginia Health System, Charlottesville, Virginia

MARY E. NORTON, MD
Professor and Interim Chair, Department of Obstetrics, Gynecology, and Reproductive Sciences, University of California San Francisco, San Francisco, California

BARBARA M. O'BRIEN, MD
Associate Professor, Department of Obstetrics, Gynecology, and Reproductive Biology, Beth Israel Deaconess Medical Center, Harvard Medical School, Boston, Massachusetts

KARI L. RING, MD, MS
Assistant Professor, Division of Gynecologic Oncology, Department of Obstetrics and Gynecology, University of Virginia Health System, Charlottesville, Virginia

BRIAN L. SHAFFER, MD
Associate Professor, Obstetrics and Gynecology/Maternal-Fetal Medicine, Oregon Health & Science University, Portland, Oregon

BLAIR K. STEVENS, MS, CGC
Department of Obstetrics, Gynecology and Reproductive Sciences, McGovern Medical School, The University of Texas Health Science Center at Houston, Houston, Texas

MELISSA STOSIC, MS
Associate Director of Reproductive Genetics, Department of Obstetrics and Gynecology, and the Institute of Genomic Medicine, Columbia University Medical Center, New York, New York

CHANTAE SULLIVAN-PYKE, MD
Fellow, Division of Reproductive Endocrinology and Infertility, Department of Obstetrics and Gynecology, University of Pennsylvania, Philadelphia, Pennsylvania

NEETA VORA, MD
Division of Maternal-Fetal Medicine, Department of Obstetrics and Gynecology, The University of North Carolina at Chapel Hill, Chapel Hill, North Carolina

RONALD WAPNER, MD
Professor, Department of Obstetrics and Gynecology, and the Institute of Genomic Medicine, Columbia University Medical Center, New York, New York

Contents

Prenatal carrier screening has expanded to include a larger number of genes and variants offered to all couples considering or with an ongoing pregnancy. Panethnic screening for cystic fibrosis and spinal muscular atrophy and screening for a limited number of conditions based on ethnicity are recommended by the American College of Obstetricians and Gynecologists. Residual risk calculations have become an obsolete part of posttest counseling when expanded carrier screening (ECS) is selected. The Perception of Uncertainties in Genome Sequencing scale offers a useful understanding of the pretest and posttest counseling concerns that should be considered as part of ECS implementation.

Preimplantation genetic testing encompasses preimplantation genetic screening (PGS) and preimplantation genetic diagnosis (PGD). PGS improves success rates of in vitro fertilization by ensuring the transfer of euploid embryos that have a higher chance of implantation and resulting in a live birth. PGD enables the identification of embryos with specific disease-causing mutations and transfer of unaffected embryos. The development of whole genome amplification and genomic tools, including single nucleotide polymorphism microarrays, comparative genomic hybridization microarrays, and next-generation sequencing, has led to faster, more accurate diagnoses that translate to improved pregnancy and live birth rates.

The clinical integration of prenatal genetic technologies raises a series of important medical and ethical considerations for patients, families, health care providers, health care systems, and society. It is critical to recognize, understand, and address these issues in conjunction with the continued development of new prenatal genetic screens and tests. This article discusses some of the lead ethical issues as a starting point to further understand their ramifications on patients, families, communities, and health care providers.

Recurrent pregnancy loss is often idiopathic, but numerical and structural chromosomal abnormalities constitute an important cause. Numerical chromosomal abnormalities in the conceptus are primarily due to meiotic nondisjunction; the rate and complexity of embryonic aneuploidy are driven by female age. Structural chromosomal abnormalities (balanced translocations or inversions) can lead to unbalanced gametes depending on specific recombination and segregation patterns during meiosis. The attendant reproductive risk depends on the type of rearrangement and its parental origin. Current methods for the analysis of products of conception include cytogenetics, array comparative genomic hybridization, and

Obstetrician gynecologists play a critical role in the identification of women who may carry a germline mutation placing them at an increased lifetime risk of gynecologic and nongynecologic cancers. Given this, all gynecologists must have a basic understanding of the most common hereditary cancer syndromes, the associated cancer risks, and possible risk-reducing interventions to play a proactive role in the care of these women. This article presents general guidelines and potential tools for identification of high-risk patients, reviews the current literature regarding genetic mutations associated with gynecologic malignancies, and proposes screening and risk-reduction options for high-risk patients.

OBSTETRICS AND GYNECOLOGY CLINICS

Foreword

Update on Reproductive Genetics: What an Obstetrician-Gynecologist Needs to Know

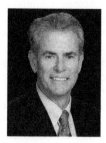

William F. Rayburn, MD, MBA
Consulting Editor

A major goal of prenatal care is to help ensure birth of a healthy infant while minimizing risk to the mother. This achievement includes the early identification and management of pregnancies at risk for early reproductive loss and later fetal morbidity and mortality. Care should be initiated as early as preconception in select cases and before the end of the first trimester, since some screening and diagnostic tests can be performed by then.

This issue of *Obstetrics and Gynecology Clinics of North America*, guest edited by Dr Lorraine Dugoff, focuses on reproductive genetics that deals with preconception, preimplantation, and early prenatal genetic counseling and screening. Reproductive genetics is a field of obstetrics that is undergoing significant change. This issue provides an excellent overview about preimplantation and prenatal genetic counseling.

Genetic abnormalities emphasized in this issue involve aneuploidy, microdeletion syndromes, and carrier screening. The American College of Obstetricians and Gynecologists (ACOG) and American College of Medical Genetics and Genomics recommend that all women be informed, ideally at the first prenatal visit, about the availability of testing options so that they can make an informed decision.

Referral to a genetic counselor is useful to discuss a specific disorder, residual risk, options for diagnosis, and reproductive alternatives after a non-reassuring finding. The complexity involved in pretest and posttest risk assessment underscores the importance of genetic counseling both before and after any testing. Key ethical issues and cost considerations are described in this issue to improve informed choices.

Two major noninvasive screening tests include maternal serum levels of specific biochemical markers and cell-free DNA in the maternal circulation. Specific biochemical markers associated with Down syndrome (trisomy 21) and trisomy 18, with or without

Obstet Gynecol Clin N Am 45 (2018) xiii–xiv
https://doi.org/10.1016/j.ogc.2017.12.002
0889-8545/18/© 2017 Published by Elsevier Inc.

ultrasound markers, may detect other fetal conditions beyond the primary targets. Noninvasive prenatal screening using cell-free DNA in the maternal circulation to screen for trisomy 21, 18, and 13 and sex chromosome aneuploidies is another acceptable approach. Furthermore, cell-free DNA testing offers the option for fetal RhD genotype screening for Rh isoimmunization cases.

Patients electing to undergo genetic screening should understand the differences between screening and diagnostic tests. Couples need to understand what can and cannot be screened, how to interpret positive and negative screen results, how to be informed about false positive and negative results, the need for any subsequent invasive or noninvasive testing, and the possible reproductive choices. Genetic analyses are performed at various commercial laboratories. More testing options, such as chromosomal microarray analysis and whole exome sequencing, as described in this issue, have become available.

The ACOG position on carrier screening is that "ethnic-specific, panethnic, and expanded carrier screening are acceptable strategies for preconception and prenatal carrier screening. Every obstetrician-gynecologist or other women's health care provider should establish a standard approach that is consistently offered to and discussed with each patient, ideally before pregnancy." After counseling, a patient may decline any carrier screening. In addition, all patients should be offered carrier screening for cystic fibrosis and spinal muscular atrophy, as well as a complete blood count and screening for thalassemias and hemoglobinopathies. If the patient is determined to be a carrier for a specific condition, her reproductive partner should be offered screening to determine the couple's risk of having an affected child.

Included in this issue is an overview about genetic screening for hereditary cancers in gynecology. The most common hereditary cause is the presence of germline mutations in the tumor suppressor genes and breast cancer type 1 and 2 susceptibility genes (*BRCA1* and *BRCA2*). In clinical practice, most women who undergo genetic testing do not have a mutation for either of these genes. Next-generation sequencing multigene panels are available to evaluate for a wider array of potential mutations. Expertise is required to ensure that the appropriate test is ordered and that the test will be adequately interpreted, so that results can positively influence management of the patient or family members at risk for hereditary cancer.

I appreciate Dr Dugoff's effort in preparing an excellent update about reproductive genetics. Her selection of authors underscores their expertise and commitment to women with specific genetic conditions. Recognizing the remarkable evolution in this field, every obstetrician-gynecologist would benefit from reading this update and using it as a reference for their team-based practice.

William F. Rayburn, MD, MBA
Continuing Medical Education & Professional Development
MSC 10 5580, 1 University of New Mexico
Albuquerque, NM 87131-0001, USA

E-mail address:
WRayburn@salud.unm.edu

Preface

Reproductive Genetics

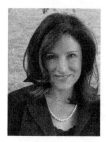

Lorraine Dugoff, MD
Editor

The rapid progress and discoveries in molecular genetics in recent years have led to an increasing number of advances in the field of reproductive genetics. Prenatal diagnosis and genetics, which was largely focused on amniocentesis and karyotype analysis for advanced maternal age, have changed significantly over the last decade with improved screening technologies resulting in a dramatic reduction in the use of diagnostic procedures. The use of chromosomal microarray technology in women undergoing invasive procedures has enhanced the ability to detect an increased number of pathogenic conditions, particularly in fetuses with structural abnormalities. Carrier screening has historically targeted a relatively small number of disorders, largely based on ethnicity. High-throughput genotyping and sequencing approaches, which allow for efficient screening of a large number of conditions simultaneously, have led to the development of expanded carrier screening panels, which may include dozens to hundreds of diseases. Similar approaches may also be used to identify patients at risk for hereditary cancer. Identification of disease-causing mutations offers opportunities to couples to eradicate transmission to future generations through preimplantation genetic diagnosis.

The rapidly advancing developments in the field of reproductive genetics may present challenges to care providers who currently offer or would like to introduce these new tests into their practices. Education of providers and patients is critical. In addition, application of new genetic technology has generated many complex ethical issues. The goal of this issue is to provide the general obstetrician-gynecologist with an overview of the advances in the field of reproductive genetics.

The authors highlighted in this issue are leaders in the field of reproductive genetics. The issue opens with an overview of genetic counseling by Jennifer Hoskovec and Blair Stevens. This is followed by several articles focused on prenatal screening and prenatal diagnosis. Drs Brian Shaffer and Mary Norton review the use of cell-free DNA screening for fetal aneuploidy, which is becoming increasingly popular and

Obstet Gynecol Clin N Am 45 (2018) xv–xvi
https://doi.org/10.1016/j.ogc.2017.12.001
0889-8545/18/© 2017 Published by Elsevier Inc.

more widely used than conventional screening with maternal serum analytes. Drs Kristin Gerson and Barbara O'Brien cover the application of cell-free DNA technology to single-gene disorders and determination of fetal RhD genotype. Dr Whitney Burns and I review the challenges and options associated with aneuploidy screening in multiple gestations. The next two articles focus on the application of newer technologies in prenatal diagnosis. Melissa Stosic and Drs Brynn Levy and Ron Wapner review the application of microarray technology, and Drs Angie Jelin and Neeta Vora cover whole-exome sequencing. We then move on to the topic of carrier screening. Drs Jennifer King and Susan Klugman review ethnicity-based carrier screening, and Dr Anthony Gregg provides an overview of expanded carrier screening. Next, Drs Chantae Sullivan-Pyke and Anuja Dokras review how the information discovered using whole-genome amplification and genomic tools is applied in preimplantation genetic screening and preimplantation genetic diagnosis to improve pregnancy outcomes and live birth rates. Drs Ruth Farrell and Megan Allyse discuss key ethical issues in prenatal genetics. This is followed by an overview on the status of genetic screening in recurrent pregnancy loss by Dr Daniel Kaser. The final article by Drs Kari Ring and Susan Modesitt highlights the information physicians should know about genetic testing, screening, and risk reduction in hereditary cancers in gynecology.

It is exciting and a bit daunting to think about the content of a future issue on reproductive genetics. It is likely that noninvasive whole-genome sequencing of the fetus and treatment and prevention of genetic abnormalities and human disease using gene editing will become available as the field of reproductive genetics continues to advance. For the time being, it is important for the practicing obstetrician-gynecologist to have an understanding of current practice as reviewed in this issue. I am most appreciative of my colleagues who presented the topics in this issue. I believe that you will find the articles to be of value and applicable to your practice.

Lorraine Dugoff, MD
Divisions of Maternal Fetal Medicine
and Reproductive Genetics
University of Pennsylvania
Perelman School of Medicine
2 Silverstein 3400 Spruce Street
Philadelphia, PA 19104, USA

E-mail address:
Lorraine.Dugoff@uphs.upenn.edu

Genetic Counseling Overview for the Obstetrician-Gynecologist

Jennifer M. Hoskovec, MS, CGC*, Blair K. Stevens, MS, CGC

KEYWORDS

- Genetic counseling • Genetics • Genetic testing • Pretest counseling
- Family history • Risk assessment • Informed consent

KEY POINTS

- This article outlines a framework for the process of genetic counseling in the primary obstetric and gynecologic setting.
- Specifics regarding risk assessment, family history evaluation, genetic testing, and pretest and posttest counseling are discussed.
- The article provides strategies for counseling patients effectively and addresses when a referral for additional genetic counseling by a specialized genetics provider should be considered.

INTRODUCTION

Genetic counseling is becoming an increasingly integral part of health care, as rapidly advancing technologies have resulted in the discovery of genetic conditions and predisposition to disease as well as a plethora of genetic testing options. Thirty million Americans are affected by a rare condition, 80% of which are caused by genetic abnormalities,[1] and these conditions are frequently encountered in the obstetric setting. Approximately 3% of all children born in the United States have a major birth defect, 20% of which have an underlying genetic etiology.[2]

In a time when discussions about genetics have become part of routine care, obstetrician-gynecologists are poised to be the initiators of genetic counseling. For many women of childbearing age, their obstetrician-gynecologist is their primary medical provider.[3] As such, the obstetrician-gynecologist is a trusted source of medical

The authors have no conflicts of interest to disclose.
Department of Obstetrics, Gynecology and Reproductive Sciences, McGovern Medical School, The University of Texas Health Science Center at Houston, 6410 Fannin Street, Suite 1217, Houston, TX 77030, USA
* Corresponding author.
E-mail address: Jennifer.E.Malone@uth.tmc.edu

Obstet Gynecol Clin N Am 45 (2018) 1–12
https://doi.org/10.1016/j.ogc.2017.10.008
0889-8545/18/© 2017 Elsevier Inc. All rights reserved.

information and women of childbearing age report that they prefer to receive genetic information from their obstetrician-gynecologist as opposed to other sources.[4]

Advancements in knowledge and technology have led to the development of thousands of genetic tests. Health care providers must understand the benefits, limitations, and utility of these various options to facilitate responsible and effective integration of genetic testing into clinical care. The American College of Obstetricians and Gynecologists (ACOG) has 17 publications addressing genetic issues, including testing, and how they should be addressed in the clinical obstetric and gynecologic setting (**Table 1**). From routine family history assessment and genetic carrier screening to caring for women with a genetic condition, these publications speak to the complexity of reproductive genetics and highlight the need for genetic counseling.

This article outlines a framework for the process of genetic counseling in the primary obstetric and gynecologic setting, provides strategies for counseling patients effectively, and addresses when a referral for additional genetic counseling by a specialized genetics provider should be considered.

Table 1
American College of Obstetricians and Gynecologists publications regarding genetics in women's care

Committee Opinion 409	Direct-to-Consumer Marketing of Genetic Testing	June 2008 Reaffirmed 2016
Committee Opinion 410	Ethical Issues in Genetic Testing	June 2008
Committee Opinion 478	Family History as a Risk Assessment Tool	March 2011 Reaffirmed 2015
Committee Opinion 488	Pharmacogenetics	May 2011 Reaffirmed 2016
Committee Opinion 527	Personalized Genomic Testing for Disease Risk	June 2012 Reaffirmed 2016
Committee Opinion 634	Hereditary Cancer Syndromes and Risk Assessment	June 2015
Committee Opinion 616	Newborn Screening and the Role of the Obstetrician-Gynecologist	January 2015 Reaffirmed 2016
Committee Opinion 640	Cell-free DNA Screening for Fetal Aneuploidy	September 2015
Committee Opinion 643	Identification and Referral of Maternal Genetic Conditions in Pregnancy	October 2015
Committee Opinion 682	Microarrays and Next-Generation Sequencing Technologies: The Use of Advanced Genetic Diagnostic Tools in Obstetrics and Gynecology	December 2016
Committee Opinion 690	Carrier Screening in the Age of Genomic Medicine	March 2017
Committee Opinion 691	Carrier Screening for Genetic Conditions	March 2017
Committee Opinion 693	Counseling About Genetic Testing and Communication of Genetic Test Results	April 2017
Practice Bulletin 103	Hereditary Breast and Ovarian Cancer Syndrome	April 2009 Reaffirmed 2017
Practice Bulletin 147	Lynch Syndrome	November 2014 Reaffirmed 2016
Practice Bulletin 162	Prenatal Diagnostic Testing for Genetic Disorders	May 2016
Practice Bulletin 163	Screening for Fetal Aneuploidy	May 2016

DEFINITION OF GENETIC COUNSELING

Genetic counseling is the communication process in which trained professionals help people understand and adapt to the medical, psychosocial, and familial implications of genetic contributions to disease. The process integrates the following:

- Interpretation of family and medical histories to assess the chance of disease occurrence or recurrence
- Education about inheritance, testing, management, prevention, resources, and research
- Counseling to promote informed choices and adaptation to the risk or condition[5]

It is important to note that although discussion of genetic testing is typically part of the genetic counseling process, it is not the goal of genetic counseling. Given the optional nature of most genetic tests, balanced and accurate information is key for patients to make informed choices that are in line with their personal values, needs, and desires.

Risk Assessment

There are several components to genetic counseling, and successful completion of each relies on proper risk assessment. Determining patients' specific risk factors allows for appropriate counseling, test selection, and test interpretation. Risk assessment entails evaluation of a patient's medical, family, pregnancy, exposure, and travel histories, as well as factors such as ethnicity and age. Assessment of the partner's medical, family, and travel history is also necessary.

Evaluating family history regularly allows for identification of patients with an increased risk for inherited genetic conditions, birth defects, hereditary cancer, and conditions with genetic predisposition, such as diabetes and mental illness. Family history collection should include details such as medical conditions, ages of onset, relation to patient, and relevant genetic testing results. Family history concerns prompting additional genetic counseling are listed in **Box 1**.[6]

Box 1
Family history concerns prompting additional genetic counseling

- Family history of known or suspected genetic condition
- Ethnic predisposition to certain genetic disorders
- Consanguinity
- Multiple affected family members with the same or related disorders
- Earlier than expected age of onset of disease
- Multifocal or bilateral occurrence of disease (often cancer) in paired organs
- One or more major malformations
- Developmental delays or intellectual disabilities
- Abnormalities in growth
- Recurrent pregnancy loss (2 or more)

Modified from the National Coalition for Health Professionals Education in Genetics: Core Principles in Family History; with permission. Available at: https://www.jax.org/education-and-learning/clinical-and-continuing-education/ccep-non-cancer-resources/core-principles-in-family-history.

Various tools can aid collection of family health information, such as patient questionnaires, online tools, or a 3-generation pedigree. Patient questionnaires can be time effective and can allow the patient to obtain more detailed information from relatives when provided before an appointment. However, they are dependent on the reliability of patient reporting and may result in misinformation or lack of patient understanding.[7] A 3-generation pedigree relies on a provider-patient conversation about family history and increases the chances of identifying genetic concerns, but requires more time and genetics knowledge.[8,9] Online tools that collect patient-provided information and aid in risk assessment may allow for more streamlined and accurate collection of family health information.[9–11] Each approach has benefits and limitations, and determining the best approach for collection of family health will depend on the nature of an individual clinic and provider.

Genetic Testing

Genetic testing may be offered as part of routine prenatal care or due to a specific risk factor, such as a positive family history or abnormal ultrasound finding. There are almost 70,000 genetic testing products available in the United States, with an average of 10 new testing products entering the market per day. For example, more than 75 different cell-free DNA (cfDNA) screening tests for trisomies 21, 18, and 13 and sex chromosome abnormalities are available on the market through 33 different laboratories. Even more abundant are the more than 400 clinically available *BRCA1* and/or *BRCA2* testing options through numerous laboratories. Determining which test product and which laboratory can be an onerous task.[12]

A clinical practice may choose to use more than 1 laboratory depending on the various testing needs, testing methodology, turnaround time, insurance type, or other patient-specific factors. Points to consider when determining which laboratory to use can be found in **Box 2**.

Once the laboratory is identified, the appropriate test must be selected. For example, cystic fibrosis testing of the *CFTR* gene may involve testing for specific mutations known to a family, a 32-mutation *CFTR* panel, an expanded *CFTR* mutation panel, or *CFTR* sequencing depending on clinical circumstances. Incorrect selection of a genetic test can result in misdiagnosis, additional costs, and delayed results.[13] Proper risk assessment, including evaluation of the family history, and an understanding of the types of genetic testing options, can aid in the correct selection of a genetic test. Genetic test selection requires varying degrees of genetics knowledge and

---

Box 2
Points to consider when selecting a genetic testing laboratory

- Test performance: Sensitivity, specificity, positive predictive value, negative predictive value, test failure rate. Are test performance metrics based on internal data or peer-reviewed data?

- Test Logistics: What are sample requirements? How are samples transported to the laboratory? Are shipping/courier services available? What is the test turnaround time?

- Test reporting: What is included on test reports? Are results clear and concise? How are abnormal results communicated to the ordering physician? Are results available online?

- Support: Are genetics experts available to providers with questions? Are genetic counseling services available to patients?

- Billing: Is laboratory in-network with insurance plans? What are self-pay prices? Are payment plans available? Is there an online price estimator? Does the laboratory offer billing support directly to the patient?

expertise depending on the test in question. When needed, the client services team or genetic counselor from the testing laboratory or a clinical genetic counselor, medical geneticist, or maternal-fetal-medicine specialist can serve as a resource in determining the best genetic test for a patient.

Pretest Counseling

Pretest counseling is an imperative component to the genetic testing process, as it enables informed decision making and informed consent. The pretest counseling process includes patient education and discussion that facilitates autonomous decision making about whether to undergo genetic testing and, if so, which test to pursue. For patients who elect testing, the anticipatory guidance delivered during pretest counseling also will aid the provider in delivering results effectively.

Pretest counseling should include information about the purpose of testing; how the test is performed; test accuracy; the benefits, risks, and limitations of testing; possible results; and implications of those results and secondary or incidental findings from testing (**Box 3**). Test performance data that are useful in the pretest counseling setting include detection rate (sensitivity) and false-positive rate (specificity). For some patients, benefits of testing can include the desire for more information and less uncertainty, more informed decision making regarding medical management, and reassurance. Limitations and risks of genetic testing may include false-positive or false-negative results, uncertainty surrounding results, stress or anxiety, and in some cases, the risk for procedure-related complications (ie, amniocentesis).

Box 3
Pretest counseling components

- What is the purpose of the test?
- How is the test performed (eg, blood test, invasive procedure)?
- How accurate is the test?
- What are the risks of testing?
  - Complications
  - Misinformation
  - Uncertain results
  - Incidental findings
  - Anxiety/stress
- What are benefits of testing?
  - Information
  - Management
  - Treatment/prevention
- What are possible results?
  - Positive
  - Negative
  - Uncertain
  - No results
- What is the turnaround time for results?
- How will results be communicated?
- Will results have implications for other family members?
- Is testing covered by insurance?
- Optional nature of testing

Individuals will weigh these risks and benefits differently and may come to different conclusions about whether to pursue testing. Therefore, the optional nature of genetic testing should be emphasized.

Adequate pretest counseling will ensure proper informed consent is obtained and this consent should be documented in the patient's medical record. Informed consent can be documented with a signed consent form or may be noted by the provider in the patient chart. Documentation is equally important for patients who decline genetic testing.

For those who proceed with testing, a plan for results disclosure, including information on turnaround time and the method of results disclosure (phone call, online, or in-person communication), should be discussed at the time of pretest counseling. Patients who decline testing should be made aware of the option to undergo testing at a later date, or lack thereof.

Counseling about expanded carrier screening demonstrates how pretest counseling can aid in posttest counseling, both for the provider and patient. There is a high likelihood that a patient will test positive as a carrier for at least 1 condition when undergoing expanded carrier screening, particularly when the larger panels, which include screening for greater numbers of conditions, are used. Informing a patient before testing that it is likely he or she will screen positive as a carrier for at least 1 condition will better prepare patients who end up with positive screen results.

Pretest genetic counseling can be performed in a variety of ways, but should be performed in a nondirective manner that is sensitive to a patient's culture, education level, language, and values. The extent and amount of pretest counseling will depend on the nature of the genetic test. If counseling aids, such as videos, online tutorials, or written information are used, a follow-up discussion is recommended to confirm patient understanding and to give the patient an opportunity to ask questions. Caution should be paid when using pretest counseling aids produced by companies performing the tests, as the information may be presented in a biased fashion. Pretest counseling can be delivered by a variety of health care providers in addition to a genetic counselor, such as an obstetrician-gynecologist, nurse practitioner, or nurse, as long as the provider has adequate knowledge of genetics and genetic testing.

Insurance coverage of genetic testing is frequently a concern for patients and may depend on several factors. Genetic testing may or may not be covered under a patient's insurance plan, and preauthorization may be required, particularly for less-routine testing. Proper risk assessment will allow for identification of a risk factor that may demonstrate medical need. Patients have a responsibility to understand their insurance plan, including deductibles and co-insurance, and providers have a responsibility to understand the medical necessity of genetic testing based on standards of care and to provide guidance in determining whether genetic testing is a covered benefit. Some laboratories have online cost estimators or billing teams that can also assist patients and providers.

In addition to insurance coverage, patients may have concerns over insurance discrimination based on a genetic test result or genetic condition. The Genetic Information Nondiscrimination Act (GINA) was signed into law in 2008 and provides protections against employer and health insurance discrimination. It is important to note that GINA protections do not apply to life insurance, disability insurance, or long-term care insurance and has exceptions such as members and family members of the US military, veterans, or individuals working for groups with 15 or fewer members.[14]

Posttest Counseling

Depending on the screening or diagnostic nature of the genetic test, normal or low-risk results often have an associated residual risk. Residual risk after a negative screening test is due to screening sensitivity of less than 100%. For example, a low-risk cell-free DNA screen for aneuploidy decreases but does not eliminate the chance for Down syndrome. Another metric that can be used to express residual risk is negative predictive value, or the chances the condition is not present given a negative result. Residual also risk can apply for conditions that are not included in a test. For example, a negative expanded carrier screening panel reduces the carrier risk for many recessive conditions, but does not assess risk for *all* genetic conditions. This residual risk should be communicated at the time of results disclosure. Although negative genetic testing results provide reassurance, the limitations should be recognized and discussed during posttest counseling as well.

The first step in posttest counseling for abnormal results is understanding what the results mean. Genetic test reports may be straightforward, but often can be confusing. Only providers with sufficient knowledge of genetics should interpret and disclose abnormal genetic test results to patients. If results are unclear, the laboratory should be contacted for more information. Many genetic testing laboratories employ genetic counselors who are able to provide more information on test results.

Delivering results that indicate an increased risk, in the case of a screening test, or an abnormal diagnostic test result should be tailored to a patient's knowledge level in an emotionally and culturally sensitive manner. When genetic testing is performed during pregnancy, results must be communicated promptly to allow for time to consider reproductive options, such as termination of pregnancy.

Disclosure of a screening result indicating an increased risk should include information about the condition, the degree of risk indicated by the results, and additional testing options, such as diagnostic testing or testing a partner. Rather than sharing information about test sensitivity or specificity, the most helpful statistical to describe abnormal screening results is the positive predictive value. Positive predictive value is the chance the condition is present given a positive result. For example, the sensitivity and specificity for cell-free DNA screening may be greater than 99% for Down syndrome, but a 23-year-old woman with an abnormal cell-free DNA result has a 50% positive predictive value, meaning her pregnancy has a 50% chance to have Down syndrome and a 50% chance to not have Down syndrome. A referral to a genetic counselor, medical geneticist, or maternal-fetal-medicine specialist should be considered for abnormal screening results.

Information to be shared about abnormal diagnostic test results include balanced and up-to-date information on the natural history of the condition, available treatment or therapies, pregnancy management options (when applicable), and available support resources. Support resources may include written or online information about the diagnosis, online or in-person support networks, state or federal aid programs, and referral to specialists. Additional information that may be appropriate to discuss immediately or at a follow-up appointment can include discussion of the etiology, recurrence risks, and testing for at-risk family members. A referral to a genetic counselor, medical geneticist or maternal-fetal-medicine specialist is encouraged for abnormal diagnostic test results.

Support

Genetic information and testing have unique characteristics that make genetic counseling and the need for patient support integral components to patient care. These characteristics include the predictive capability of genetic testing, uncertainty surrounding certain types of results, the impact on other family members, and the evolving knowledge and interpretation of genetic information.[15] Genetic counseling is a process that involves an exchange of information and avenue for patient education. In addition to this exchange, the genetic counseling process provides an opportunity for a provider to explore a patient's values, desires, and needs. Understanding patient needs allows for personalized care and emotional support. Genetic counseling and testing often can be accompanied by emotions such as uncertainty and anxiety. Addressing these emotional needs, both before and after testing, or supporting the decision to not undergo testing, is key to high-quality patient care. When a patient understands information, and feels heard and supported by his or her provider, it promotes patient satisfaction, recall, autonomy, and compliance.[16]

Although short-term support is provided during genetic counseling and routine obstetric and gynecologic care, some patients may require longer-term support. Several indications frequently encountered in the obstetric and gynecologic clinic, such as miscarriage, fetal genetic diagnoses, termination of pregnancy, or cancer diagnoses, often carry a heavy emotional toll that may require additional referrals and/or support. Referral information for local grief therapists and mental health counselors, support networks (in person or online), and written information can be helpful resources for patients during these trying times.

GENETIC COUNSELING IN CLINICAL PRACTICE

Genetic counseling may be provided by various medical professionals, including obstetrician-gynecologists. However, given the complexity of the information, those who provide genetic counseling should have expertise in the field of medical genetics, knowledge of the benefits, limitations and utility of genetic testing, and infrastructure for counseling and referral.

Training in genetics for obstetrician-gynecologists is extremely variable across residency programs. The Council on Resident Education in Obstetrics and Gynecology's Educational Objectives is a framework intended to guide obstetrics and gynecology residency curriculum development. The following are the objectives outlined for "Genetics"[17]:

1. Solicit a family pedigree
2. Describe and perform preconception counseling and testing
3. Describe and perform antepartum counseling and testing
   - Perform prenatal screening
   - Refer for diagnostic testing

These objectives are broad, leaving significant room for flexibility in the development of genetics curriculum for each obstetrics and gynecology residency program. On one hand, this is beneficial, because the specifics of genetic testing in the obstetrics and gynecology setting is ever-changing, as evidenced by the number of new and updated college committee opinions on these topics (see **Table 1**). However, there is significant potential for gaps in education, particularly with regard to the complexity of the technologies, the clinical utility and interpretation of results, and the applicability of these tests to broad populations of patients. Finally, the need for continuing education on genetics topics is imperative for practicing obstetrician-gynecologists to maintain competent knowledge of genetic testing.

In a busy clinical practice, it can be challenging to determine the most effective way to incorporate genetic counseling and testing and there is no one-size-fits-all approach. The ultimate goal is to offer the right test, to the right person, at the right time in their care while promoting informed decision making. Potential barriers to implementation include, but are not limited to, time constraints, adequate staffing, genetics expertise, and concerns regarding insurance coverage of testing options.

Genetic Counseling Models

Depending on the variables in any given clinic, there are multiple models for incorporating genetic counseling and testing that may be considered:

1. Primary counseling provided by the obstetrician-gynecologist. The obstetrician-gynecologist completes the risk assessment, provides genetic counseling, and facilitates routine genetic screening/testing. Referral to a genetic specialist may be indicated for patients meeting specific criteria. Examples of referral indications may include, but are not limited to the following[18]:
   - Age 35 years or older at the time of delivery (singleton pregnancy)
   - Age 33 years or older at the time of delivery (twin pregnancy)
   - Close blood relative of her partner (consanguinity)
   - Abnormal first or second trimester maternal serum screen
   - Exposure to teratogen during gestation
   - Fetal anomaly on ultrasound or echocardiogram
   - Personal or family history of pregnancy complications associated with genetic factors
   - Positive carrier screen for genetic condition
   - Personal history of stillbirth or recurrent pregnancy loss
   - Family history of genetic condition, birth defect, intellectual disabilities, hearing loss, or vision loss
   - Either member of the couple with a chromosome abnormality
   - Family history of cancer or cancer known to be associated with specific genes
   - Mental illness, such as schizophrenia, depression, or bipolar disorder
2. Primary counseling provided by the obstetrician-gynecologist in conjunction with supplementary counseling resources, including interactive online tutorials, online resources, or written materials. There are a variety of professionally developed resources aimed at helping obstetrician-gynecologists educate patients about the various genetic testing options. Although this is not a supplement for a family history assessment and an individualized conversation regarding decision making, these tools can help provide patient-centered information about prenatal genetic testing. Organizations such as the ACOG, Society for Maternal Fetal Medicine, National Society of Genetic Counselors, American College of Medical Genetics and Genomics, and Perinatal Quality Foundation have a variety of society-guided resources that may meet the needs for some obstetrics and gynecology practices. A referral to a genetic specialist still may be considered for the indications listed previously.
3. Primary counseling provided by a genetic counselor. Some practices with readily available access to genetic counselors may use the genetic counselor as the primary provider of all genetic counseling discussions, including routine testing options.

When primary genetic counseling is provided by an obstetrician-gynecologist, the following steps should be considered:

1. Determine how risk assessment will be obtained
2. Determine the appropriate testing options for each patient population (average risk and increased risk) and when testing options will be discussed
3. Determine the best laboratory (or laboratories) for your patient population
4. Determine the best approach for results disclosure
5. Develop triage model for referral to genetic specialist, as indicated

Collaborative Care

Genetic counselors have long worked in conjunction with obstetrician-gynecologists, often as part of a maternal-fetal medicine service. In a recent professional survey, 67% of genetic counselors providing direct patient care reported receiving referrals from obstetrician-gynecologists.[19] The obstetrics and gynecology specialty continues to move toward a more comprehensive model for women's care with a patient-centered collaborative approach. This shift includes incorporating other health care professionals into the care model to improve efficiency and increase patient satisfaction.[3] Genetic counselors are poised to work with obstetrician-gynecologists in a collaborative model by serving as a resource for genetic expertise, both for physicians and their patients.

Certified Genetic Counselors (CGCs) are professionals with specialized training in medical genetics and counseling who receive board certification through the American Board of Genetic Counseling. The Accreditation Council for Genetic Counseling outlines 22 practice-based competencies that must be demonstrated by an entry-level genetic counselor to practice. Similar to the CREOG (Council on Resident Education in Obstetrics and Gynecology) learning objectives for obstetrics and gynecology residency programs, these practice-based competencies are a guide for a genetic counseling training program curriculum as well as the development of the board certification examination. These competencies are divided into the following 4 domains:

1. Genetics expertise and analysis
2. Interpersonal, psychosocial, and counseling skills
3. Education
4. Professional development and practice

As outlined in the National Society of Genetic Counselors Scope of Practice, the responsibilities of a genetic counselor are threefold: (1) to provide expertise in clinical genetics; (2) to counsel and communicate with patients on matters of clinical genetics; and (3) to provide genetic counseling services in accordance with professional ethics and values.[20]

Today there are nearly 4000 CGCs in the United States, working in a variety of clinical, research, and industry settings. Approximately 80% of CGCs providing direct patient care work in the prenatal or cancer genetics setting.[19] Although most genetic counselors in direct patient care provide one-on-one, face-to-face counseling in a university medical center or hospital setting, alternative delivery models, such as group counseling, phone counseling, and telemedicine, are being used more frequently to increase access to patient care.

Genetic testing laboratories often employ genetic counselors who can serve as a resource for medical professionals with regard to testing specifics and results interpretation. Additionally, some laboratories offer posttest genetic counseling via phone for patients who have questions regarding their results.

SUMMARY

Genetic counseling is a process that should be embedded into the obstetrics and gynecology practice as a part of routine care. The particular model used will vary among practices and should be implemented with patient population, provider expertise, clinic resources, and infrastructure in mind. Pretest counseling is essential to ensuring patient autonomy, informed decision-making, and quality patient care. Although the basics of prenatal genetic counseling and testing may be effectively facilitated in the general obstetrics and gynecology setting, a triage model to identify patients who would benefit from additional genetic counseling from a specialty provider, such as a CGC or medical geneticist, is a necessary component to a comprehensive care approach.

REFERENCES

1. RARE diseases: facts and statistics. Global Genes 2017. Available at: https://globalgenes.org/rare-diseases-facts-statistics/. Accessed June 26, 2017.
2. Martin JA, Hamilton BE, Osterman MJ, et al. Births: final data for 2015. Natl Vital Stat Rep 2017;66(1):1.
3. Rayburn WF, Tracy EE. Changes in the practice of obstetrics and gynecology. Obstet Gynecol Surv 2016;71(1):43–50.
4. Mandelberger AH, Robins JC, Buster JE, et al. Preconception counseling: do patients learn about genetics from their obstetrician gynecologists? J Assist Reprod Genet 2015;32(7):1145–9.
5. National Society of Genetic Counselors' Definition Task Force, Resta R, Biesecker BB, et al. A new definition of genetic counseling: National Society of Genetic Counselors' Task Force report. J Genet Couns 2006;15(2):77–83.
6. American College of Obstetricians and Gynecologists Committee on Genetics. Committee opinion no. 478: family history as a risk assessment tool. Obstet Gynecol 2011;117(3):747–50.
7. St Sauver JL, Hagen PT, Cha SS, et al. Agreement between patient reports of cardiovascular disease and patient medical records. Mayo Clin Proc 2005;80(2): 203–10.
8. Hafen LB, Hulinsky RS, Simonsen SE, et al. The utility of genetic counseling prior to offering first trimester screening options. J Genet Couns 2009;18(4):395–400.
9. Doerr M, Teng K. Family history: still relevant in the genomics era. Cleve Clin J Med 2012;79(5):331–6.
10. Edelman EA, Lin BK, Doksum T, et al. Implementation of an electronic genomic and family health history tool in primary prenatal care. Am J Med Genet C Semin Med Genet 2014;166C(1):34–44.
11. Wu RR, Myers RA, McCarty CA, et al. Protocol for the "implementation, adoption, and utility of family history in diverse care settings" study. Implement Sci 2015;10:163.
12. The current landscape of genetic testing. 2017. Available at: https://www.concertgenetics.com/wp-content/uploads/2017/05/10_ConcertGenetics_Current LandscapeofGeneticTesting_2017Update.pdf. Accessed June 27, 2017.
13. Miller CE, Krautscheid P, Baldwin EE, et al. Genetic counselor review of genetic test orders in a reference laboratory reduces unnecessary testing. Am J Med Genet A 2014;164A(5):1094–101.
14. Genetic Non-Discrimination Act of 2008, 122 Stat. 881 (2008).
15. McGuire AL, Fisher R, Cusenza P, et al. Confidentiality, privacy, and security of genetic and genomic test information in electronic health records: points to consider. Genet Med 2008;10(7):495–9.
16. Meiser B, Irle J, Lobb E, et al. Assessment of the content and process of genetic counseling: a critical review of empirical studies. J Genet Couns 2008;17(5): 434–51.
17. Blanchard MH, Robinson RD, Brewer MA, et al. Educational Objectives: core curriculum in obstetrics and gynecology. 11th Edition. American College of Obstetrics and Gynecologists; 2016. Available at: https://www.acog.org. Accessed June 15, 2017.
18. Pletcher BA, Toriello HV, Noblin SJ, et al. Indications for genetic referral: a guide for healthcare providers. Genet Med 2007;9(6):385–9.

19. National Society of Genetic Counselors: 2016 Professional Status Survey Executive Summary. (2016, May). Available at: http://www.nsgc.org/page/whoaregeneticcounselors. Accessed June 15, 2017.
20. Genetic counselors' scope of practice. Available at: http://genetics.emory.edu/gc_training/documents/NSGC%20Scope%20of%20Practice.pdf. Accessed June 6, 2017.

Cell-Free DNA Screening for Aneuploidy and Microdeletion Syndromes

Brian L. Shaffer, MD[a],*, Mary E. Norton, MD[b]

KEYWORDS

- Prenatal screening • Cell-free DNA screening • Noninvasive prenatal testing
- Aneuploidy screening • Prenatal diagnosis

KEY POINTS

- Cell-free DNA screening has high detection rates for the most common fetal autosomal and sex chromosomal aneuploidies, but should not be considered diagnostic.
- Positive predictive value (PPV) should be used in counseling women after a positive cell-free DNA screen; diagnostic testing should be offered for confirmation and is strongly recommended before termination.
- Cell-free DNA screening is available for some microdeletions, but due to a low prevalence and therefore a low PPV, should not be used in the general population until clinical validation studies indicate value in the low-risk obstetric patient.
- Cell-free DNA screening is less accurate due to confined placental mosaicism and with twins, and may lead to incidental findings, such as maternal copy number variants (CNVs), mosaicism, and maternal cancer.
- Nondirective pretest education and counseling should be provided with emphasis on the potential benefits, risks, and limitations before cell-free DNA screening.

INTRODUCTION

The use of cell-free DNA (cfDNA) in aneuploidy screening and prenatal genetic testing is rapidly evolving. This test has been called a "disruptive innovation," a term used to describe innovations that displace existing technologies with something generally more efficient and worthwhile.[1] cfDNA screening is a far more effective screening test for Down syndrome than current multiple marker screening with serum analytes

---

Disclosure Statement: B.L. Shaffer has nothing to disclose. M.E. Norton has received research support from Natera.
[a] Obstetrics and Gynecology/Maternal-Fetal Medicine, Oregon Health Sciences University, 3181 SW Sam Jackson Park Road, L458, Portland, OR 97239, USA; [b] Department of Obstetrics, Gynecology, and Reproductive Sciences, University of California, San Francisco, Box 0132, 550 16th Street, 7th Floor, San Francisco, CA 94143, USA
* Corresponding author.
E-mail address: shaffer@ohsu.edu

Obstet Gynecol Clin N Am 45 (2018) 13–26
https://doi.org/10.1016/j.ogc.2017.10.001
0889-8545/18/© 2017 Elsevier Inc. All rights reserved.

and nuchal translucency ultrasound.[2,3] However, it is more expensive than current screening, and does not detect as many chromosome abnormalities as invasive diagnostic testing, especially if chromosomal microarray is used.[4] It also cannot provide information about the range of conditions that can be suspected based on multiple marker screening.[5]

Some laboratories have added testing for chromosomal microdeletions to their cfDNA panels. Pathogenic chromosomal microdeletions or microduplications (copy number variants or CNVs) overall occur in approximately 1% of fetuses and newborns.[4] However, this number refers to all possible CNVs in a population, whereas cfDNA screening typically tests for only 4 or 5 such disorders. Although the well-recognized 22q11.2 microdeletion syndrome included on cfDNA panels is relatively common, affecting approximately 1 of 4000 to 5000 individuals,[6] most others are far less common with incidences closer to 1 of 30 to 50,000. Such testing has not been validated in clinical studies, rather validation studies have included mixing of normal and abnormal DNA in laboratory samples.[7] Even with very high sensitivity and specificity, at such low prevalence, the positive predictive value (PPV) of such testing is likely very low and the clinical utility is unclear.

WHAT IS CELL-FREE DNA AND HOW IS IT USED FOR SCREENING?

cfDNA consists of small (50–200 base pairs) fragments of DNA that circulate in the maternal plasma. Fetal cfDNA originates from the trophoblast after apoptosis and after 10 weeks of gestation accounts for approximately 10% to 15% of the total cfDNA in the maternal serum.[8–10] Because the fetus and placenta are almost always identical, cfDNA can therefore be used to screen for fetal genetic disorders. cfDNA screening is also known as cfDNA testing, NIPT (Noninvasive Prenatal Testing), and NIPS (Noninvasive Prenatal Screening) and requires accurate quantification of DNA from a specific chromosome to determine the probability of fetal chromosomal abnormalities.

Different laboratories use various techniques and bioinformatics analyses to estimate the probability of a fetal chromosome abnormality. Massively parallel shotgun sequencing (MPSS) is a technique in which millions of cfDNA fragments are amplified, sequenced, and mapped to each chromosome based on a unique sequence. By counting a massive number of fragments, fetal and maternal DNA does not need to be separated and the relative proportion of each chromosome (maternal and placental) can be compared with a reference and a risk for aneuploidy can be calculated.[11,12] Because of the complex and resource-intensive nature of MPSS, other techniques have been developed to sequence and count only selected regions of chromosomes of interest, called chromosome selective sequencing (CSS). CSS uses polymerase chain reaction to amplify segments unique to chromosomes 13, 18, 21, and the sex chromosomes, thus reducing the workload and (potentially) the relative cost of screening without sacrificing performance. Finally, an odds ratio (OR) is generated using the individual a priori risk, and the chromosome counts accounting for the fetal fraction (FF).[8,13] Another technique for screening with cfDNA takes advantage of single nucleotide polymorphisms (SNPs) on specific chromosomes of interest. DNA from maternal leukocytes is separated from the maternal plasma, which contains both maternal and fetal cfDNA. Differences among informative SNPs in the maternal sample, cfDNA, and a reference sample (or paternal, if available) can be compared via a complex informatics algorithm to provide a risk for aneuploidy. SNP-based techniques are less prone to amplification variation and can theoretically detect triploidy as well as uniparental disomy (UPD). In addition to differences in how the sequencing and laboratory analyses are performed, there are also differences in the bioinformatics analysis and interpretation.[14,15]

The interpretation and presentation of results from each laboratory are important and complex aspects of understanding and comparing the overall test characteristics. Regardless of the laboratory technique or method of reporting, most clinical tests are done to screen for fetal chromosomal disorders, including trisomy 13, 18, and 21, as well as differences of sex chromosomes, although some laboratories provide testing for other trisomies (eg, trisomies 9, 16, and 22) and selected microdeletion syndromes (eg, 22q11.2 deletion, 4p minus) using the techniques described previously.[16,17]

PERFORMANCE OF CELL-FREE DNA SCREENING FOR COMMON AUTOSOMAL TRISOMIES

cfDNA is used to screen for the common fetal aneuploidies (ie, 13, 18, and 21) and sex chromosomal abnormalities; the accuracy for each of these varies somewhat by condition and platform used.[3,7,9,14,18]

Trisomy 21

In a recent meta-analysis of 30 studies and more than 225,000 pregnancies, the detection rate of cfDNA for trisomy 21 was 99.7% (95% confidence interval [CI] 99.1–99.9), whetrsd the false-positive rate was 0.04% (95% CI 0.02%–0.08%).[18] Individual studies also compare cfDNA with traditional serum and ultrasound-based screening (eg, sequential or integrated screening), which has a detection rate of approximately 90%, a screen positive of approximately 4%, and a PPV of 6%[19] **(Table 1)**. The detection rate, however, should not be confused with the probability that the fetus is affected given a positive screening result, known as the PPV. Some cfDNA laboratories report only that a result is "positive," together with the accompanying sensitivity (eg, 99%), which some clinicians have inappropriately interpreted as a 99% chance that the fetus is affected. Reporting without a PPV implies a degree of certainty that is diagnostic or near diagnostic. Indeed, the detection rate of greater than 99% applies only to the women successfully screened (ie, who obtain a result), and not an individual patient's risk.

Following a positive result, women should be counseled about the posttest probability (or PPV) that the fetus has the disorder in question; conversely, if a result returns low risk or negative, then the negative predictive value (NPV) or the probability

Table 1
Performance of cell-free DNA screening for common aneuploidy and sex chromosome aneuploidy

Condition	Detection, %	False Positive, %	Positive LR	Negative LR
Trisomy 21	99.7	0.04	2509	0.003
Trisomy 18	98.2	0.05	2330	0.022
Trisomy 13	99.0	0.04	2819	0.010
Monosomy X	95.8	0.14	694	0.042
Other SCA[a]	100	0.004		

Abbreviations: LR, likelihood ratio; SCA, sex chromosome aneuploidy.
[a] Other SCA: 47, XXX; 47, XXY; 47, XYY.
Adapted from Gil MM, Accurti V, Santacruz, B, et al. Analysis of cell-free DNA in maternal blood in screening for aneuploidies: updated meta-analysis. Ultrasound Obstet Gynecol 2017;50(3):302–14; with permission.

that the fetus is not affected should be used in posttest counseling. In studies of a general obstetric screening population, the PPV for cfDNA screening following an abnormal Down syndrome result ranges from 45% to 76%.[3,8,9] Of note, some patients (6.2%) have been reported to terminate a pregnancy after a positive cfDNA screen without diagnostic testing, highlighting the need for pretest and posttest education and counseling, as well as confirmation of a cfDNA screen with a diagnostic test.[20]

cfDNA testing must be considered *screening* despite PPVs for trisomy 21 that have been reported at greater than 90%. In a recent study of primary aneuploidy screening in a general pregnancy population, the PPV was 75% for trisomies, including 13, 18, and 21.[21] Using the a priori risk, which may be based on maternal age or a specific risk after traditional screening, an individual PPV can be calculated. The authors recommend an online calculator to assist obstetric providers in counseling their patients using both PPV and NPV (https://www.perinatalquality.org/vendors/nsgc/nipt/).

Trisomies 13 and 18

Although these conditions are considerably less common than Down syndrome, cfDNA screening for trisomies 13 and 18 also has high detection rates for both trisomy 18 (98.2%, CI 95.5%–99.2%) and trisomy 13 (99.0%, CI 65.8%–100%). cfDNA screening for these trisomies also has low false-positive rates. Larger CIs around the detection rate for trisomy 13 is due to the lower prevalence compared with trisomies 18 and 21[18] (see **Table 1**).

Monosomy X (Turner Syndrome)

All major cfDNA screening laboratories offer the option for sex determination (ie, presence of Y) or to assess for sex chromosome aneuploidy (SCA), but these data are considerably more sparse. Indeed, 11 published studies accounting for a total of only 36 cases of monosomy X were included in a recent meta-analysis. The pooled weighted detection rate for monosomy X by cfDNA screening was 95.8% (95% CI 70.3%–99.5% with a false-positive rate of 0.14% (95% CI 0.05%–0.08%). Associated likelihood ratios of 694 are incorporated into online calculators and can provide positive predictive value after a test result indicating monosomy X or a PPV of approximately 40% (given that the prevalence of this condition varies little with maternal age) can be used to assist in counseling and decision making regarding diagnostic testing.

Other Sex Chromosome Aneuploidies

Most laboratories offering cfDNA screening will allow patients and their providers to select or "opt in" for SCA screening (eg, 47XXY, 47XXX, 47XYY). Compared with monosomy X, these data are even more limited and should be interpreted with some caution. Further, clinicians should be aware that a positive cfDNA screen for 47, XYY may actually be confirmed on diagnostic testing to be 47, XXY. Although these conditions are both sex chromosome aneuploidies, Klinefelter syndrome (47, XXY) has a considerably different and more severe phenotype compared with the expected outcomes of those with 47 XYY, again emphasizing the screening nature of this test and the importance of diagnostic confirmation. Nonetheless, reported detection rates are high; however, clinicians should realize that PPVs and NPVs may not be accurately determined depending on the predicted SCA.[18]

CHROMOSOMAL MICRODELETIONS

Some laboratories also provide cfDNA screening for a select number of microdeletions. Pathogenic chromosomal microdeletions or microduplications, also known as CNVs, are associated with a significant risk of cognitive disability and/or long-term medical issues. More than 40 well-known deletion and duplication syndromes have been well delineated, and although penetrance and expressivity may vary, all have important clinical and developmental consequences. These CNVs have, in general, a similarly severe phenotype to the other conditions for which prenatal screening is routinely provided and, as such, testing for them is of interest to patients and clinicians alike.

The well-described microdeletion syndromes, such as Prader-Willi syndrome, are individually much less common than Down syndrome, although across the genome CNVs occur in more than 1% of fetuses and newborns.[4] Although many microdeletion syndromes have important clinical consequences, most cfDNA microdeletion screening panels currently include only 5 to 6 specific disorders with a combined prevalence of approximately 1 of 2500. In addition to the limited number of conditions included on most clinical panels, molecular microdeletions may account for only a proportion of those individuals with a given clinical phenotype. For instance, the deletion causing Prader-Willi syndrome accounts for only 65% to 75% of cases, whereas the remainder are caused by UPD or a single gene change, neither of which would be detected on cfDNA screening.[22] The most prevalent of these conditions is the 22q11.2 deletion syndrome; most cases result from a 3 MB deletion on chromosome 22. However, this relatively large deletion is estimated to account for approximately 87% of disease-causing deletions, whereas the remainder are caused by a considerably smaller deletion that is unlikely to be detected by cfDNA screening.[23] Thus, a significant proportion of these clinical cases would not be detected; therefore, even if the sensitivity for the larger deletion is very high, the sensitivity for the clinical disorder is likely far lower, although data are extremely limited. Despite a negative test, the disorder cannot be ruled out by cfDNA screening.

The low baseline prevalence of each of these microdeletion syndromes significantly limits the PPV, which will therefore be much lower than that achieved in screening for the common trisomies. The PPV is likely to be fairly similar to that reported with traditional serum screening for aneuploidy. cfDNA screening for microdeletions has not been studied in large clinical trials and, as such, data on PPV are limited. One study with follow-up of 61 positive cfDNA microdeletion screens reported a PPV of 17%.[7] More recently, investigators from a single high-volume center reported on all of the abnormal cfDNA microdeletion results over more than 2 years; of note, a large proportion of women were referred for abnormal screening results or ultrasound abnormalities. Of the 16 positive cfDNA screens for a microdeletion, 12 had diagnostic testing with microarray and 0 of 12 were found to carry a fetus with a microdeletion syndrome (PPV 0%), casting doubt on the clinical utility cfDNA screening for microdeletions.[24] Thus, women who desire testing for CNVs, or who prefer comprehensive testing for as many disorders as possible, should be offered diagnostic testing with chromosomal microarray. Given these data, the American College of Obstetricians and Gynecologists (ACOG) and the Society for Maternal-Fetal Medicine conclude that routine screening for microdeletions with cfDNA is not recommended.[25,26]

FETAL CELL-FREE DNA CONTRIBUTION, OR FETAL FRACTION

Fetal cfDNA can be detected in the maternal serum reliably by approximately 9 weeks of pregnancy and increases throughout gestation, with considerably more fetal cfDNA present in the maternal serum after 20 weeks. Fetal cfDNA is cleared quickly after delivery with levels undetectable by 2 hours after delivery.[10,27,28] The FF is the proportion of the total cfDNA that is derived from the fetus/placenta and an important variable in the accuracy of cfDNA screening; in fact, the most common reason for test failure (approximately 50%) is due to too little fetal DNA being present, or a low FF. An FF of 3.5% to 4.0% is the lower limit of fetal DNA needed for accurate detection of fetal aneuploidy.[3,11] Several biologic factors can influence the fetal fraction. As suggested previously, FF is typically too low before 10 weeks for reliable cfDNA screening. In addition, as maternal weight increases, the FF decreases. In one study, the FF was reported to be less than 4% in approximately 7% of women who weigh $\geq$100 kg, whereas women weighing more than 160 kg had an approximately 50% risk of having low FF.[29] In addition to low FF, inappropriate sample collection or treatment can lead to the inability to test the sample, also resulting in a failed result. Samples are usually collected in an EDTA tube and centrifuged within a short time of collection to prevent the maternal white blood cells from degrading and diluting the fetal component. Increased no-call results due to a low FF also have been associated with anticoagulation with enoxaparin (adjusted OR 37.5, 11.19–125.87, P<.0001).[30] Finally, the platform used may impact test failure rates, which have been reported to be more common in SNP-based approaches (6.4%) when compared with MPSS platforms (1.6%).[31]

Certain aneuploidies (particularly trisomy 18 and triploidy) have been associated with a lower FF and the potential for test failure, therefore a "no-call" result has implications beyond lost time to gain information about the pregnancy, as this is associated with an increased risk of fetal aneuploidy. Specifically, in samples that were analyzed and a result was not provided, a recent meta-analysis determined that the chance for a common aneuploidy was 5.9%, whereas the risk was 11.7% for SCA.[18] In another study, the OR for aneuploidy was 9.2 in cases with failed cfDNA tests.[32] Considering these risks, women whose serum is sent for cfDNA screening and no result is obtained should be counseled about the risks of aneuploidy, particularly increased risks of trisomy 13, 18, and triploidy, and offered diagnostic testing. For women who decline diagnostic testing, repeat cfDNA testing can be expected to provide a result in a subsequent sample in 50% to 80% of cases.[33,34]

FALSE POSITIVES AND INCIDENTAL FINDINGS

There are limitations to the accuracy of cfDNA screening for common aneuploidies due to some relatively common biologic variables and complications of pregnancy, including multiple gestations, vanishing twins, and confined placental mosaicism. At present, there are limited data on cfDNA screening for aneuploidy in multifetal gestations; most studies have included only a small number of fetuses with aneuploidy. In fact, a recent large meta-analysis included studies with a combined total of 24 cases of trisomy 21, 14 of trisomy 18, and a single case of trisomy 13.[18]

The detection rate of cfDNA screening for Down syndrome in the setting of a multiple gestation is high but the failure rate has been reported to be greater than with singletons due to a low FF.[35–37] Further, cfDNA screening also may lead to a false positive in the setting of a vanishing twin, as a high proportion of fetal losses are due to aneuploidy, and the surviving co-twin will most often be unaffected. With few data available, PPV cannot currently be calculated in such a situation, and if cfDNA is used in a known (or unknown) twin gestation, individualized counseling is required. Routine screening for aneuploidy using cfDNA in multifetal gestations is therefore not recommended given these limitations and the limited data.[25,26]

Confined placental mosaicism (CPM) is identified in 1% to 2% of pregnancies based on results of chorionic villus sampling, and can lead to a false-positive cfDNA screen. Because the trophoblastic tissue of the placenta is the primary source of fetal cfDNA, this may lead to a positive cfDNA due to placental aneuploidy in the setting of a healthy fetus. From a clinical and patient-centered perspective, this represents a false-positive result given that the fetus is chromosomally normal; however, laboratories may consider this analytically correct, as there is additional aneuploidy material in the cfDNA. Again, this highlights the importance of the recommendation that a positive cfDNA screening result should be confirmed with diagnostic testing. It has been argued that diagnostic follow-up of a positive cfDNA result should preferentially be done via amniocentesis, given the potential that a positive result may represent CPM and therefore chorionic villus sampling (CVS) may return a mosaic result requiring further clarification. However, for a patient early in gestation, given the high PPV of cfDNA and the high possibility of a true-positive result, there are advantages to the earlier confirmation provided by CVS.[38]

A number of maternal chromosomal abnormalities may lead to discordant cfDNA screening results and incidental findings. Low-level maternal mosaicism (eg, 46XX/45X)[39] or maternal 47,XXX[40] has been associated with false-positive cfDNA screening results for SCA. Some have proposed performing a maternal karyotype in cases with a false-positive cfDNA for fetal sex chromosomal aneuploidy (particularly 45,X or 47,XXX) to assess for maternal mosaicism.[41] Others have reported that maternal CNVs, including partial duplication of chromosomes 13, 18, or 21, may account for up to 10% of false-positive cfDNA screens.[42,43] Positive cfDNA screens also can be caused by maternal unbalanced rearrangements. Single gene duplications can likewise be identified by cfDNA screening, and these have been reported to be associated with disorders leading to late-onset visual loss, hematologic abnormalities, including thrombocytopenia and myeloid malignancy,[44] and familial, early-onset Alzheimer disease.[45]

Maternal malignancy has been reported in the setting of a positive screening result, particularly in cases with multiple genetic abnormalities identified, in which additional material from 1 or more chromosomes and/or missing material of others is identified by cfDNA screening. A small proportion of DNA screening tests (0.03%) may result in such chaotic findings, and in 1 report, 18% of women were found to have malignancy, including leukemia, lymphoma, and colorectal cancer, when multiple abnormalities were present by cfDNA screening.[46] Given that cfDNA screening is not intended to screen for maternal cancer or CNVs that predispose to medical issues, such as thrombocytopenia or early-onset Alzheimer disease, caution is warranted. In the context of the limitations of short-term and long-term outcome data, associated costs and burden of a potential workup, as well as the potential anxiety given possibly risk for malignancy, it remains unclear what testing should be used when false-positive results are identified.

PRETEST COUNSELING

Given the potential for false-positive or false-negative results, the high risk of an abnormal outcome with a positive result (PPV), and the possibility of incidental findings, it is important that pretest education and counseling include mention of these potential outcomes. Discussions regarding options for prenatal testing for aneuploidy should occur before any screening or testing, and typically occur in the context of the first prenatal care visit. Specific components of genetic counseling include pretest education, counseling, and informed consent; indeed, the core of genetic counseling is to determine patient preferences and expectations, and there is consensus that such genetic counseling should be *nondirective*.

Prenatal care is provided by several different practitioners with different backgrounds, knowledge, and skill in discussing the components of screening for aneuploidy with cfDNA. This discussion may be held by a midwife, nurse practitioner, family practitioner, generalist obstetrician, or perinatologist; in other settings, education by telemedicine or a group presentation by a genetic counselor are used. Regardless of the setting or the specific provider, the difference between screening and diagnostic tests should be discussed, as well as the fact that cfDNA is a screening test that detects a limited number of chromosomal abnormalities.[47] This is particularly important because a considerable proportion of women interviewed (13%–40%) after cfDNA counseling and testing answered that there was "no chance" of fetal Down syndrome after a negative result.[21,48] Patients should understand that screening tests are noninvasive tests that provide risk estimates, whereas diagnostic tests are invasive tests that provide a certain diagnosis. Key to the discussion is the baseline or a priori risk of a fetal abnormality and the factors that may contribute to such a risk, such as maternal age, family history, and underlying maternal medical conditions that may impact the fetal risk for a birth defect.

The pregnant woman should understand what condition(s) the test screens for, and that women opt for screening for different reasons (eg, reassurance or consideration of termination for an abnormal result). In addition, counseling should include the consequences of a positive screen, including the potential for a recommendation of a diagnostic test with an associated risk of a loss in the setting of an abnormal result. Some women may prefer to avoid screening altogether, to avoid the anxiety of a positive result knowing she would never choose to undergo a diagnostic test. In the setting of cfDNA testing, the benefits include the high detection of the common aneuploidies and monosomy X in singleton pregnancies. The limitations include the low PPV for other conditions (particularly microdeletions) if those are chosen, the possibility for a false negative and/or false positive, including incidental maternal abnormalities, such as a maternal CNV or a result that indicates an increased risk for a malignancy (**Box 1**).

Box 1
Components of pretest counseling for cell-free DNA (cfDNA) aneuploidy screening

- cfDNA screening appears to be the most accurate screening test for trisomy 21.
- cfDNA does not screen for all chromosomal conditions.
- Women who desire definitive information about chromosome conditions in their pregnancy should be offered the option of amniocentesis or chorionic villus sampling (CVS).
- False-positive and false-negative results do occur with cfDNA.
- Diagnostic confirmation with CVS or amniocentesis is recommended for women with abnormal cfDNA results.
- A negative cfDNA result indicates a decreased risk and does not definitively rule out trisomy 21 or other chromosome conditions.
- All genetic screening is elective. Whether a woman chooses to have aneuploidy screening, prenatal diagnostic testing, or no testing is a personal decision and any of these is a reasonable option.

From Society for Maternal-Fetal Medicine (SMFM) publications committee. #36: prenatal aneuploidy screening using cell free DNA. Am J Obstet Gynecol 2015;212(6):713; with permission.

INDICATIONS FOR cfDNA SCREENING

The Society for Maternal-Fetal Medicine currently recommends that cfDNA aneuploidy screening should not be routine for the general obstetric population, but only in those at increased risk for fetal aneuploidy. Specifically, women 35 years or older at delivery, those with a history of prior pregnancy with a trisomy detectable by cfDNA screening, or those with a parental balanced Robertsonian translocation with increased risk of fetal trisomy 13 or 21. Other indications include ultrasound findings indicating an increased risk of aneuploidy (ie, trisomies 13, 18, or 21) and those with a positive screen on traditional serum screening (eg, sequential screen).[26] The American College of Medical Genetics (ACMG) recommends that all pregnant women be informed of the availability of clinically relevant CNVs and does not limit cfDNA testing for the common trisomies to patients with only an increased risk for fetal aneuploidy. cfDNA genome-wide screening for microdeletions or other autosomal trisomies is not recommended by either organization.[49]

In women who opt for screening for aneuploidy, several strategies have been proposed for the general obstetric population:

1. cfDNA as a universal screening test together with first-trimester ultrasound
2. cfDNA as a second-tier screening test in which women with a positive traditional screen are offered cfDNA
3. A contingent strategy in which women at low risk (approximately 1 in <2500) by traditional screen have no additional testing, those at high risk (approximately ≥1 in 100) are offered diagnostic testing, and those at moderate risk (1 in 101–2500) are offered cfDNA.[50–53]

These strategies attempt to maximize the prenatal diagnosis of trisomies 21, 18, and 13 and minimize procedure-related losses and cost. Although these strategies maximize detection of common aneuploidies, they fail to account for other significant chromosomal abnormalities that are detected when women opt for diagnostic testing after an abnormal sequential/integrated screen.

COMPARISON OF CELL-FREE DNA TO TRADITIONAL SCREENING

cfDNA screening has higher detection, PPV, and NPV and lower false-positive rates compared with traditional screening for the common trisomies (ie, trisomies 13, 18, and 21); cfDNA also has good detection and PPV for SCA. In addition, cfDNA has a lower screen positive rate than traditional screening and its use has led to lower utilization of diagnostic testing.[51] However, diagnostic testing after a positive sequential or integrated screen will identify other important karyotype abnormalities in a considerable proportion of cases. Therefore, when looking at the entire cohort of screened women, given fewer diagnostic tests, and a failure to diagnose chromosome abnormalities other than the common aneuploidies, as well as the considerable number (0.8%–8%) of failed cfDNA tests (which are associated with a significantly increased risk for aneuploidy),[32] the superior performance of cfDNA on a population level is not as clear. This has prompted some investigators to compare detection of all chromosome abnormalities with sequential/integrated screening with those detected by cfDNA.

In a study of more than 450,000 women who underwent sequential screening in California, the detection rate for all chromosomal abnormalities was 81.6% with a false-positive rate of 4.5%. Further, it was estimated that cfDNA would have detected only 70% to 75% of these abnormalities[5] (Table 2). In a separate analysis of data from the California Prenatal Screening program that included more than 1.3 million women, of

Table 2
Comparison of prenatal screening and diagnostic testing options for fetal aneuploidy

Test	DR T21, %	DR All Aneuploidies, %	Screen Positive Rate[a]
First trimester screen	80	69	5
Sequential/Integrated screen	93	82	5
Cell-free DNA screen	99	72	1–9
Chorionic villus sampling	>99	>99	1[b]
Amniocentesis	>99	>99	0.2[b]

Abbreviation: DR, detection rate.
[a] Includes all results that required further follow-up (ie, failed cfDNA tests and false-positive results).
[b] Mosaicism, which includes confined placental mosaicism.
From Society for Maternal-Fetal Medicine (SMFM) Publications Committee. #36: prenatal aneuploidy screening using cell free DNA. Am J Obstet Gynecol 2015;212(6):714; with permission.

all chromosomal abnormalities that were identified by traditional aneuploidy screening followed by diagnostic testing, 16.9% would not have been detected had cfDNA analysis been performed instead of CVS or amniocentesis. In women who had positive serum screening, it was estimated that after a normal cfDNA screen, the residual risk of a chromosomal abnormality was 1 in 50, or 2%.[54] The detection rate in this study was inversely associated with maternal age; the lowest detection rate for cfDNA occurred in women younger than 25 because the relative proportion of chromosomal abnormalities other than trisomy 21, 18, or 13 is greater in younger women. These data should be used to determine not only ideal population-based but individually based screening strategies.

Indeed, when comparing 6 different screening strategies (including cfDNA screening, sequential screening, diagnostic testing, and other combinations) in a decision analytical model taking into account pregnancy outcomes, cost, and maternal utilities, sequential screening with the option for diagnostic testing in all women younger than 38 years provided the highest detection rate, optimized maternal quality adjusted life years (QALYs) and was cost saving. cfDNA screening had the best detection for trisomy 21 and maximized QALYs in women older than 38, but had lower detection for other important chromosome abnormalities. These data support the recommendation that traditional screening should be considered the optimal strategy for most women, whereas cfDNA as a primary screen should be limited to those of advanced maternal age when the relative proportion of detected aneuploidy is highest.[55]

CELL-FREE DNA IN THE OVERALL CONTEXT OF ALL CONGENITAL DISORDERS

To understand the impact of cfDNA screening on detection of clinically important congenital disease, it is important to understand the relative contribution of each type of disorder. Congenital structural malformations account for nearly 50% of congenital disease whereas the second largest component of congenital disease (approximately 24%) is due to CNVs (ie, microdeletions and duplications) that would be detected by chromosomal microarray (CMA). Single gene disorders account for approximately 15% of significant congenital diseases, with autosomal recessive disorders (9%) accounting for the largest proportion. Chromosomal abnormalities account for just more than 10% of congenital disease and approximately 80% to

85% of those are due to the common trisomies (trisomy 13, 18, and 21), as well as the sex chromosome aneuploidies. Therefore, in ideal circumstances, cfDNA screening for aneuploidy would be expected to detect, at best, 10% of congenital disease.

SUMMARY

cfDNA screening is an outstanding test for detection of Down syndrome, and the value of such screening is particularly apparent as maternal age increases. Indeed, the risk for aneuploidy and specifically, Down syndrome, increases considerably after age 40, whereas the risk of a significant CNV remains constant regardless of maternal age. In fact, a microdeletion syndrome is actually more likely than Down syndrome for all women younger than 40.[56] The chance of a clinically relevant CNV by CMA in the setting of a normal karyotype is approximately 1 in 60 regardless of maternal age, and is considerably higher (approximately 1 in 17) in the setting of a structural malformation.[4] ACOG recommends that all women should be offered diagnostic testing to assess for chromosome abnormalities, as no screening is expected to detect all clinically significant copy number variations. In those who opt for diagnostic testing, CMA is recommended in those with a fetal structural malformation.[57] Given that CMA detects a significant chromosome abnormality in approximately 1.7% of fetuses, and that cfDNA screens for only the common aneuploidies, cfDNA as a primary screening test would be expected to detect only approximately 12% of diagnosable chromosome abnormalities.

Expanded panels including trisomies 9, 16, and 22, as well as panels that include 5 to 10 CNVs, are unlikely to significantly increase the yield of cfDNA screening despite good detection rates. Individually, microdeletion syndromes are rare and accounting for the 6 most commonly included on cfDNA panels would result in a prevalence of approximately 1 in 2500 in a general screening population. As discussed previously, the clinical utility of cfDNA screening is limited, and recent experience suggests screening for microdeletions with cfDNA has a low PPV.[58]

Clearly, cfDNA screening has had tremendous impact on the field of prenatal diagnosis. Although this technology has provided an exciting advance in the field, at present the coverage of genomic abnormalities is far less than can be detected with diagnostic testing, particularly when chromosomal microarray is used. The field continues to advance at a rapid pace, however, with the introduction of screening for large CNVs across the genome,[59] as well as testing for single gene mutations.[60]

REFERENCES

1. Christensen CM. The innovator's dilemma: when new technologies cause great firms to fail. Boston: Harvard Business School Press; 1997. ISBN 978-0-87584-585-2.
2. Bianchi DW, Parker RL, Wentworth J, et al. DNA sequencing versus standard prenatal aneuploidy screening. N Engl J Med 2014;370(9):799–808.
3. Norton ME, Jacobsson B, Swamy GK, et al. Cell-free DNA analysis for noninvasive examination of trisomy. N Engl J Med 2015;372(17):1589–97.
4. Wapner RJ, Martin CL, Levy B, et al. Chromosomal microarray versus karyotyping for prenatal diagnosis. N Engl J Med 2012;367:2175–84.
5. Norton ME, Baer RJ, Wapner RJ, et al. Cell-free DNA vs. sequential screening for the detection of fetal chromosomal abnormalities. Am J Obstet Gynecol 2016; 214:727.e1-6.
6. Shprintzen RJ. Velo-cardio-facial syndrome: 30 years of study. Dev Disabil Res Rev 2008;14:3–10.

7. Wapner RJ, Babiarz JE, Levy B, et al. Expanding the scope of noninvasive prenatal testing: detection of fetal microdeletion syndromes. Am J Obstet Gynecol 2015;212:332.e1-9.

8. Norton ME, Brar H, Weiss J, et al. Non-Invasive Chromosomal Evaluation (NICE) Study: results of a multicenter prospective cohort study for detection of fetal trisomy 21 and trisomy 18. Am J Obstet Gynecol 2012;137(2):e1–8.

9. Lo YMD, Corbetta N, Chamberlain PF, et al. Presence of fetal DNA in maternal plasma and serum. Lancet 1997;350(9076):485–7.

10. Wang E, Batey A, Struble C, et al. Gestational age and maternal weight effects on cell free fetal DNA in maternal plasma. Prenat Diagn 2013;33(7):662–6.

11. Palomaki GE, Kloza EM, Lambert-Messerlian GM, et al. DNA sequencing of maternal plasma to detect Down syndrome: an international clinical validation study. Genet Med 2011;13(11):913–20.

12. Bianchi DW, Platt LD, Goldberg JD, et al, Maternal Blood is Source to Accurately Diagnose Fetal Aneuploidy (MELISSA) Study Group. Genome-wide fetal aneuploidy detection by maternal plasma DNA sequencing. Obstet Gynecol 2012;119:890–901.

13. Sparks AB, Struble CA, Wang ET, et al. Noninvasive prenatal detection and selective analysis of cell-free DNA obtained from maternal blood: evaluation for trisomy 21 and trisomy 18. Am J Obstet Gynecol 2012;206(4):319.e1-9.

14. Zimmermann B, Hill M, Gemelos G, et al. Noninvasive prenatal aneuploidy testing of chromosomes 13, 18, 21, X, and Y, using targeted sequencing of polymorphic loci. Prenat Diagn 2012;32(13):1233–41.

15. Dar P, Shani H, Evans MI. Cell-free DNA: comparison of technologies. Clin Lab Med 2016;36(2):199–211.

16. Zhao C, Tynan J, Ehrich M, et al. Detection of fetal subchromosomal abnormalities by sequencing circulating cell-free DNA from maternal plasma. Clin Chem 2015;61(4):608–16.

17. Pescia G, Guex N, Iseli G, et al. Cell-free DNA testing of an extended range of chromosomal anomalies: clinical experience with 6,388 consecutive cases. Genet Med 2017;19(2):169–75.

18. Gil M, Accurti V, Santacruz B, et al. Analysis of cell-free DNA in maternal blood in screening for aneuploidies: updated meta-analysis. Ultrasound Obstet Gynecol 2017;50:302–14.

19. Malone FD, Canick JA, Ball RH, et al, First- and Second-Trimester Evaluation of Risk (FASTER) Research Consortium. First-trimester or second-trimester screening, or both, for Down's syndrome. N Engl J Med 2005;353:2001–11.

20. Dar P, Curnow KJ, Gross SJ, et al. Clinical experience and follow-up with large scale single-nucleotide polymorphism-based noninvasive prenatal aneuploidy testing. Am J Obstet Gynecol 2014;211:527.e1-17.

21. Palomaki GE, Kloza EM, O'Brien BM, et al. The clinical utility of DNA-based screening for fetal aneuploidy by primary obstetrical care providers in the general pregnancy population. Genet Med 2017;19:778–86.

22. Driscoll DJ, Miller JL, Schwartz S, et al. Prader-Willi syndrome [Updated 2016 Feb 4]. In: Pagon RA, Adam MP, Ardinger HH, et al, editors. GeneReviews® [Internet]. Seattle (WA): University of Washington; 1998. p. 1993–2017. Available at: https://www.ncbi.nlm.nih.gov/books/NBK1330/.

23. Shaikh TH, Kurahashi H, Saitta SL, et al. Chromosome 22-specific low copy repeats and the 22q11.2 deletion syndrome: genomic organization and deletion endpoint analysis. Hum Genet 2000;9(4):489–501.

24. Valderramos SG, Rao RR, Scibetta EW, et al. Cell-free DNA screening in clinical practice: abnormal autosomal aneuploidy and microdeletion results. Am J Obstet Gynecol 2016;215:626.e1–10.

25. American College of Obstetricians and Gynecologists. Screening for fetal aneuploidy ACOG Practice Bulletin: No 163. Obstet Gynecol 2016;127:e123–37.

26. Society for Maternal-Fetal Medicine (SMFM) Publications Committee. #36: Prenatal aneuploidy screening using cell free DNA. Am J Obstet Gynecol 2015;212: 711–6.

27. Lo YM, Zhang J, Leung TN, et al. Rapid clearance of fetal DNA from maternal plasma. Am J Hum Genet 1999;64:218e24.

28. Hui L, Vaughan JI, Nelson M. Effect of labor on postpartum clearance of cell-free fetal DNA from the maternal circulation. Prenat Diagn 2008;28:304e8.

29. Ashoor G, Syngelaki A, Poon LCY, et al. Fetal fraction in maternal plasma cell-free DNA at 11-13 weeks' gestation: relation to maternal and fetal characteristics. Ultrasound Obstet Gynecol 2013;41:26–32.

30. Burns W, Koelper N, Barberio A, et al. The association between anticoagulation therapy, maternal characteristics and a failed cfDNA test due to a low fetal fraction. Prenat Diagn 2017. [Epub ahead of print].

31. Yaron Y. The implications of noninvasive prenatal testing fares: a review of an under discussed phenomenon. Prenat Diagn 2016;36:391–6.

32. Pergament E, Cuckle H, Zimmermann B, et al. Single-nucleotide polymorphism-based noninvasive prenatal screening in a high-risk and low-risk cohort. Obstet Gynecol 2014;124(2 Pt 1):210–8.

33. Sago H, Sekizawa A, Japan NIPT Consortium. Nationwide demonstration project of next-generation sequencing of cell-free DNA in maternal plasma in Japan: one-year experience. Prenat Diagn 2015;35:331–6.

34. Willems PJ, Dierickx H, Vandenakker ES, et al. The first 3,000 non-invasive prenatal tests (NIPT) with the harmony test in Belgium and the Netherlands. Facts Views Vis Obgyn 2014;6:7–12.

35. del Mar Gil M, Quezada MS, Bregant B, et al. Cell-free DNA analysis for trisomy risk assessment in first-trimester twin pregnancies. Fetal Diagn Ther 2014;35: 204–11.

36. Bevilacqua E, Gil MM, Nicolaides KH, et al. Performance of screening for aneuploidies by cell-free DNA analysis of maternal blood in twin pregnancies. Ultrasound Obstet Gynecol 2015;45:61–6.

37. Canick JA, Kloza EM, Lambert-Messerlian GM, et al. DNA sequencing of maternal plasma to identify Down syndrome and other trisomies in multiple gestations. Prenat Diagn 2012;32:730–4.

38. Mardy A, Wapner RJ. Confined placental mosaicism and its impact on confirmation of NIPT results. Am J Med Genet C Semin Med Genet 2016;172(2):118–22.

39. Wang Y, Chen Y, Tian F, et al. Maternal mosaicism is a significant contributor to discordant sex chromosomal aneuploidies associated with noninvasive prenatal testing. Clin Chem 2014;60:251–9.

40. Yao H, Zhang L, Zhang H, et al. Noninvasive prenatal genetic testing for fetal aneuploidy detects maternal trisomy X. Prenat Diagn 2012;32(11):1114–6.

41. Bianchi DW, Parsa S, Bhatt S, et al. Fetal sex chromosome testing by maternal plasma DNA sequencing: clinical laboratory experience and biology. Obstet Gynecol 2015;125:375–82.

42. Snyder MW, Simmons LE, Kitzman JO, et al. Copy-number variation and false positive prenatal aneuploidy screening results. N Engl J Med 2015;372(17): 1639–45.

43. Zhou X, Sui L, Xu Y, et al. Contribution of maternal copy number variations to false-positive fetal trisomies detected by noninvasive prenatal testing. Prenat Diagn 2017;37(4):318–22.
44. Brison N, Van Den Bogaert K, Dehaspe L, et al. Accuracy and clinical value of maternal incidental findings during noninvasive prenatal testing for fetal aneuploidies. Genet Med 2017;19(3):306–13.
45. Meschino WS, Miller K, Bedford HM. Incidental detection of familial APP duplication: an unusual reason for a false positive NIPT result of trisomy 21. Prenat Diagn 2016;36:382–4.
46. Bianchi DW, Chudova D, Sehnert AJ, et al. Noninvasive prenatal testing and incidental detection of occult maternal malignancies. JAMA 2015;314(2):162–9.
47. American College of Obstetricians and Gynecologists. ACOG Practice Bulletin. No. 77: Screening for fetal chromosomal abnormalities. Obstet Gynecol 2007; 109:217–27.
48. Piechan JL, Hines KA, Koller DL, et al. NIPT and informed consent: an assessment of patient understanding of a negative NIPT result. J Genet Couns 2016; 25:1127–37.
49. Gregg AR, Skotko BG, Benkendorf JL, et al. Noninvasive prenatal screening for fetal aneuploidy, 2016 update: a position statement of the American College of Medical Genetics and Genomics. Genet Med 2016;18(10):1056–65.
50. Nicolaides KH, Syngelaki A, Ashoor G, et al. Noninvasive prenatal testing for fetal trisomies in a routinely screened first-trimester population. Am J Obstet Gynecol 2012;207:374.e1–6.
51. Hui L, Hyett J. Noninvasive prenatal testing for trisomy 21: challenges for implementation in Australia. Aust N Z J Obstet Gynaecol 2013;53(5):416–24.
52. Gil MM, Revello R, Poon LC, et al. Clinical implementation of routine screening for fetal trisomies in the UK NHS: cell free DNA test contingent on results from first trimester combined test. Ultrasound Obstet Gynecol 2016;47:45–52.
53. Chetty S, Garabedian MJ, Norton ME. Uptake of noninvasive prenatal testing (NIPT) in women following positive aneuploidy screening. Prenat Diagn 2013; 33:542–6.
54. Norton ME, Jelliffe-Pawlowski LL, Currier RJ. Chromosome abnormalities detected by current prenatal screening and noninvasive prenatal testing. Obstet Gynecol 2014;124:979–86.
55. Kaimal AJ, Norton ME, Kuppermann M. Prenatal testing in the genomic age. Obstet Gynecol 2015;126(4):737–46.
56. Snijders RJM, Sundberg K, Holzgreve W, et al. Maternal age- and gestation-specific risk for trisomy 21. Ultrasound Obstet Gynecol 1999;13(3):167–70.
57. American College of Obstetricians and Gynecologists. The use of chromosomal microarray analysis in prenatal diagnosis. Committee Opinion No. 581. Obstet Gynecol 2013;122:1374–7.
58. Gross SJ, Stosic M, McDonald-McGinn DM, et al. Clinical experience with single nucleotide polymorphism based noninvasive prenatal screening for 22q11.2 deletion syndrome. Ultrasound Obstet Gynecol 2016;47(2):177–83.
59. Lefkowitz RB, Tynan JA, Liu T, et al. Clinical validation of a noninvasive prenatal test for genomewide detection of fetal copy number variants. Am J Obstet Gynecol 2016;215(2):227.e1–16.
60. Allen S, Young E, Bowns B. Noninvasive prenatal diagnosis for single gene disorders. Curr Opin Obstet Gynecol 2017;29(2):73–9.

Cell-Free DNA

Screening for Single-Gene Disorders and Determination of Fetal Rhesus D Genotype

Kristin D. Gerson, MD, PhD, Barbara M. O'Brien, MD*

KEYWORDS

- Prenatal diagnosis • cfDNA • Noninvasive prenatal testing • Single-gene disorders
- Prenatal screening • Rhesus D genotype

KEY POINTS

- The use of cell-free DNA (cfDNA) for diagnosis of single-gene disorders is an evolving technology, and its application is limited at this time.
- The limitations of cfDNA technology are most notable in clinical settings involving X-linked and autosomal recessive conditions, in part because background maternal mutant alleles greatly outnumber those of fetal origin.
- Examples of single-gene disorders where cfDNA has been used include rhesus D genotyping, skeletal dysplasias, congenital adrenal hyperplasia, and β-thalassemia.
- Patients undergoing prenatal diagnosis for evaluation for single-gene testing should undergo invasive testing.
- Determination of fetal rhesus D genotype with cfDNA is highly accurate with sensitivities above 99% and very low false-negative rates.

INTRODUCTION

The introduction of cell-free DNA (cfDNA) into the prenatal arena in 2011 has revolutionized prenatal screening for fetal aneuploidy. The use of cfDNA is also being investigated in the use of screening for single-gene disorders. The phenotypes of conditions caused by single-gene disorders are highly variable and depend on the specific gene location as well as the amount of genetic material that is duplicated or deleted. The use of expanded carrier screening panels will result in an increased number of couples identified at risk for having an offspring affected with a single-gene disorder. Family history may influence an individual's predisposition to single-gene disorders. Advanced paternal age is associated with an increased risk of de novo dominant

Disclosure Statement: The authors report no disclosures.
Department of Obstetrics, Gynecology, and Reproductive Biology, Beth Israel Deaconess Medical Center, Harvard Medical School, Boston, MA 02215, USA
* Corresponding author.
E-mail addresses: bmobrien@bidmc.harvard.edu; barbaramobrienmd@gmail.com

single-gene mutations, including achondroplasia, neurofibromatosis, Marfan syndrome, osteogenesis imperfect, and Apert syndrome. X-linked disorders associated with advanced paternal age in the maternal grandfather include fragile X, hemophilia B, and Duchenne muscular dystrophy. Experts advise that patients should undergo invasive testing for prenatal diagnosis of single-gene disorders. This article provides an overview of the status of cfDNA screening for single-gene disorders as well as an overview of the use of cell-free DNA in rhesus D (RhD) genotyping.

CELL-FREE DNA

During pregnancy, placental tissue undergoes continuous turnover of the villous trophoblast, thereby releasing apoptotic debris and cfDNA into the maternal circulation. Although cfDNA is often referred to as fetal, the genetic material derives from the placenta and circulates in the maternal plasma as short random genomic DNA fragments of 150 to 200 base pairs.[1–4] The fetal fraction or percentage of circulating DNA that is contributed by the fetus, is 3% to 13% of total cfDNA in the maternal circulation.[5,6] The fetal fraction increases with gestational age and is undetectable within hours after delivery.[7]

Identification of cfDNA in the maternal serum prompted a robust scientific investigation into its origin and potential clinical applications.[8–12] Noninvasive prenatal testing or cfDNA screening subsequently evolved as a powerful screening tool for the common autosomal and sex chromosome aneuploidies.

Screening Technology and Reporting

Various methodologies for analysis of cfDNA screening include massively parallel shotgun sequencing, targeted massively parallel sequencing, and single-nucleotide polymorphism–based approaches.[13–16] The technology uses cfDNA to screen for fetal aneuploidies. Overall, the detection rate for cfDNA screening for aneuploidy is 99.4% with a false-positive rate of 0.16%.[17] All modalities carry a high sensitivity and specificity rate for trisomy 21 and 13. A recent meta-analysis reported pooled detection rates for trisomy 21 at 99.7% with a false-positive rate of 0.04%.[18] Similarly, pooled detection rates for trisomy 13 were cited at 99.0% with a false-positive rate of 0.04%. For trisomy 18, however, these rates were slightly lower with a pooled detection rate of 97.9% with a false-positive rate of 0.04%.

Reporting of results can vary depending on laboratory, with some reporting risk as positive or negative, whereas others cite specific risk of aneuploidy using a numeric value. Positive and negative predictive values, however, are apt to be more meaningful from a clinical standpoint and depend on the prevalence of the condition in the screened population; higher disease prevalence results in higher positive predictive value. When applied to aneuploidy screening, positive predictive values are higher among older women given the increasing prevalence of the trisomic aneuploidies with maternal age. On this basis, the American College of Obstetricians and Gynecologists (ACOG) and the Society for Maternal-Fetal Medicine recommend that all cfDNA screening results include report of positive predictive and residual risk values.[6]

Occasionally, test results are indeterminate. Such no call results may occur in the setting of a low fetal fraction, aneuploidy, maternal obesity, treatment with low-molecular-weight heparin, or states of high cell turnover, or consanguinity.[19–23] Although low fetal fraction may be attributed to early gestational age, it has also been associated with pregnancies affected by aneuploidy; rates of aneuploidy among patients with indeterminate results have been reported as high as 23%.[24] Thus, a no call result warrants further genetic counseling, sonographic evaluation, and possible diagnostic testing.

Limitations of Cell-Free DNA

Despite its use as a powerful screening tool, cfDNA screening is not without limitations. Some studies report lower overall detection rates of karyotypic abnormalities using cfDNA screening among low-risk patients when compared with traditional serum screening.[25] cfDNA is not a substitute for karyotype, because current use in screening for aneuploidy is limited to trisomies 13, 18, and 21 and sex chromosome aneuploidies. Confined placental mosaicism, molar or vanishing twin pregnancies, and abnormalities arising from maternal cfDNA, including malignancy, may also confound interpretation of results.[26–29]

Given the limitations of cfDNA and the paucity of data on cost-effectiveness among low-risk women, ACOG advises conventional screening methods as first line for low-risk women.[6] The American College of Medical Genetics and Genomics recommends informing patients that cfDNA is the most sensitive screening modality for the detection of fetal aneuploidies, even among low-risk women.[30] Both governing bodies recommend that women select the screening approach that aligns most closely with their personal preferences.

Pretest counseling is critical, because the positive predictive value and negative predictive value depend on both the sensitivity of the screening test in addition to the prevalence of the aneuploidy within the population.[31] Patients must be counseled that results of cfDNA screening depend on their pretest risk of aneuploidy. Other important pretest counseling points include review of the optional nature of testing, definition of screening, clinical features and variability of conditions, and limitations to current technology.[32]

SINGLE-GENE DISORDERS

Single-gene disorders occur as a result of DNA changes at a single-gene locus. Also known as mendelian or monogenic disorders, these genetic alterations result in various disease conditions and manifest through predictable inheritance patterns. They represent a more significant proportion of genetic diseases compared with chromosomal abnormalities. Recent carrier screening data from a cohort of more than 350,000 individuals suggests that severe monogenic disorders may affect between 0.1% and 0.4% of all pregnancies.[33] Other reports cite the global prevalence of single-gene disorders to be approximately 1%.[34] Often parents are aware of their increased pregnancy risk because their own carrier status is known prior to conception. The increasing use of expanded carrier screening is likely to increase this knowledge.

Advanced paternal age has been linked to increased risk of de novo monogenic disorders, in particular those arising from mutations at the FGFR2, FGFR3, and RET genes.[35] These genetic mutations result in conditions including Pfeiffer syndrome, Crouzon syndrome, Apert syndrome, achondroplasia, thantophoric dysplasia, multiple endocrine neoplasia types 2A and 2B. One study estimated the risk of autosomal dominant disorders to be as high as 0.5% among children born to fathers of advanced paternal age; however, subsequent studies suggest that the risk is actually lower.[36,37] The risk of X-linked disorders, such as Duchenne muscular dystrophy and hemophilia, has been associated with increased age of maternal grandfather at the time of maternal birth.[38,39]

Prenatal diagnosis of single-gene disorders has historically relied on invasive methodologies, including amniocentesis and chorionic villus sampling (CVS). ACOG quotes a 1/900 risk of loss from amniocentesis and a 1/400 risk of loss from CVS.[40] In addition to associated risk of miscarriage, these tests are unable to be performed until 11 weeks' gestation. cfDNA, in contrast, can be detected at 5 weeks' gestation and can be used reliably for screening purposes by 9 weeks' to 10 weeks' gestation.[41] Thus, this modality theoretically offers safer and earlier testing compared with traditional methods.

In addition to aneuploidy screening and sex determination, cfDNA technology has been applied to prenatal detection of fetal blood group systems as well as diagnosis of autosomal dominant, autosomal recessive, and X-linked disorders (**Table 1**). cfDNA techniques used for the detection of single-gene disorders require more sophisticated approaches than those used for aneuploidy screening. The use of cfDNA for diagnosis of single-gene disorders is an evolving technology, and its application is limited at this time. Some researchers promote the concept that, in contrast to aneuploidy screening where positive results necessitate further invasive testing to confirm a diagnosis, cfDNA testing for single-gene disorders may be considered diagnostic; thus, amniocentesis or CVS is not required as follow-up. This argument is based on the premise that placental mosaicism and maternal chromosomal abnormalities are unlikely to have an impact on or confound results in this context.[42–44] As such, the technology is often referred to as noninvasive prenatal diagnosis.

The use of cfDNA in the diagnosis of single-gene disorders carries the potential to inform medical decision making with respect to surveillance and management of pregnancies at known risk for severe conditions.[45] This technology may lessen the need for invasive testing, thereby reducing the risk associated with such procedures from both an obstetric and psychological standpoint. Moreover, screening for monogenic

Table 1 Conditions diagnosed using cell-free DNA	
Aneuploidy	Trisomy 21 Trisomy 18 Trisomy 13 Turner syndrome XXX Klinefelter syndrome XYY
Blood group systems	Rh Kell
Autosomal dominant disorders[a]	Achondroplasia Thanatophoric dysplasia Apert syndrome Myotonic dystrophy Huntington disease
Autosomal recessive disorders[a]	Cystic fibrosis Congenital adrenal hyperplasia Sickle cell anemia β-Thalassemia Spinal muscular atrophy Gaucher disease Wilson disease
X-linked recessive disorders[a]	Hemophilia Duchenne muscular dystrophy Becker muscular dystrophy

[a] Examples are included but not limited to these conditions.

disorders using cfDNA may permit early intervention in pregnancies that require fetal treatment to prevent disease progression, including metabolic disorders and congenital malformations.[46–48]

Concerns regarding the use of cfDNA in the diagnosis of single-gene disorders include costs of testing as well as the potential for disparities in access among women of low socioeconomic groups. Many of these genetic diseases are rare and require individualized testing approaches developed on a family-specific basis.[49] In some countries, screening low-risk pregnancies for more common pathogenic de novo autosomal dominant mutations may become available. This practice may be extended to autosomal recessive and X-linked diseases as technologies evolve. Sequencing of maternal DNA in addition to cfDNA will likely be necessary and contribute to overall cost. Given the low prevalence of many of these monogenic disorders, validation may prove challenging and require invasive testing to confirm diagnoses until larger studies can be conducted over time.[49] As technologies evolve, ethical concerns may also arise related to informed consent, pressure to undergo testing, and decisions surrounding termination.[50–55]

AUTOSOMAL DOMINANT DISORDERS

Applications of cfDNA screening in single-gene disorders include testing for autosomal dominant mutations that occur de novo or are paternally inherited; such approaches avoid the complicating effects of maternal cfDNA. Detection of these disorders follows a logic similar to gender determination, wherein characteristics of the fetus are identified that are unique from the maternal genetic background. Specifically, fetal gender determination can be accomplished through identifying the presence of absence of Y chromosome–specific sequences, such as DYS14 or SRY.[12] Technological advances in digital PCR and DNA next-generation sequencing (NGS) have made it possible to discriminate affected from unaffected fetuses in cases, including those involving inheritance of a maternal mutant maternal allele.[56]

Amicucci and colleagues[57] examined a role for cfDNA in diagnosis of myotonic dystrophy, an autosomal dominant disorder with unstable CTG expansion on the myotonic dystrophy kinase (DMPK) gene, and demonstrated ability to identify CTG-expanded DMPK alleles in the maternal serum using PCR technologies. Chitty and colleagues[56] examined assays for analysis of cfDNA in prenatal diagnosis in skeletal dysplasias involving de novo mutations of the fibroblast growth factor receptor 3 (FGFR3) gene and highlighted a potential role for NGS in providing accurate and sensitive diagnosis of achondroplasia and thanatophoric dysplasia. Similar approaches have been applied effectively to Huntington disease and early onset primary dystonia I.[58,59]

Several commercial laboratories in the United States and United Kingdom offer commercially available noninvasive screening to individual families at risk of paternally inherited autosomal dominant or recessive conditions, advertising this modality as diagnostic for monogenic conditions and replacing invasive prenatal testing.[44] Some companies now offer an advanced paternal age panel for the diagnosis of autosomal dominant and X-linked disorders. One American commercial laboratory currently provides a panel that screens for 25 conditions.[60] Although the detection rate for screened conditions is reported at greater than 99%, the prevalence of these disorders is low in the general population, and thus these commercially offered tests are not well validated. A second company offers testing for a variety of monogenic disorders, although no validation data has been published to date.[61] In the United Kingdom, a UK National Health Service regional genetics laboratory offers noninvasive prenatal testing for autosomal dominant and de novo conditions as well as paternal exclusion of autosomal recessive disorders.[62] Use of cfDNA to test for autosomal recessive disorders does, however, requires more sophisticated technology and is not considered routine at this time. A majority of the tests are performed using NGS, which is generally a better diagnostic approach for such conditions.[50]

X-LINKED AND AUTOSOMAL RECESSIVE CONDITIONS

cfDNA has also been used to screen for paternal mutations when parents carry different mutations for autosomal recessive conditions, such as congenital adrenal hyperplasia and cystic fibrosis.[50,63,64] When cfDNA is used for this application, invasive testing is required for definitive diagnosis to assess whether the maternal mutation has also been inherited. With respect to congenital adrenal hyperplasia, a vast majority of cases arise as a result of a deficiency in 21-hydroxylase, an enzyme involved in the synthesis of glucocorticoids and mineralocorticoids. Antenatal steroid therapy may be used to suppress accumulation of androgenic metabolic precursors, thus preventing in utero virilization of an affected female fetus; treatment is not indicated for male fetuses. cfDNA screening has been used to stratify treatment need based on gender; however, traditional platforms do not permit prenatal exclusion of unaffected female fetuses. Chiu and colleagues[63] applied polymerase chain reaction (PCR) technologies to further differentiate pregnancies with affected versus nonaffected female fetuses on the premise that the unaffected female fetus express the wild-type paternally inherited allele detectable in maternal serum. Distinguishing between maternal and paternal origin was achieved through amplification of 2 paternal alleles after HLA haplotyping.

The limitations of cfDNA technology are most notable in clinical settings involving X-linked and autosomal recessive conditions, in part because background maternal mutant alleles greatly outnumber those of fetal origin.[13,65] For example, determining whether a male fetus is affected by an X-linked condition for which the mother is a known carrier requires more sophisticated technology, because the presence of the genetic mutation in maternal plasma may be of maternal or fetal origin. The same challenge applies to autosomal recessive conditions in which both parents carry the same mutation. Another common scenario involves the presence of a paternally inherited autosomal recessive mutation in the maternal serum, necessitating further testing to determine whether the fetus is affected (homozygote) or unaffected (heterozygote).

RELATIVE MUTATION DOSING AND EVOLVING TECHNOLOGIES

Such challenges may be overcome using a digital PCR-based approach called relative mutation dosage, which takes into consideration the dosage ratio of mutant to wild-type alleles in maternal serum. Lun and colleagues[66] used this technology to β-thalassemia to identify pregnancies in which the fetus was an affected homozygote in the setting of the mother being a heterozygous carrier. The assay involves a statistical model called the sequential probability ratio test, which screens for the presence of allelic imbalance based on expected ratios of maternal to fetal cfDNA. To overcome challenges associated with low levels of circulating fetal cfDNA, enhanced efficiency is achieved through a molecular enrichment strategy called digital nucleic acid size selection, which serves to increase the fetal fraction of DNA at loci of interest. The same technology was thereafter applied to other autosomal recessive diseases, including sickle cell anemia, as well as X-linked disorders, such as hemophilia.[67,68] A similar approach involves high-throughput linked-read sequencing followed by maternal plasma-based relative haplotype dosage analysis, thus bypassing the need for

DNA information from affected family members.[69] Hudecova and colleagues[70] have applied this strategy to prenatal screening for thalassemias.

Additional cfDNA technologies include haplotype-based NGS, droplet digital PCR, minisequencing, bespoke/targeted NGS, coamplicifaction at lower denaturation temperature PCR and microarray, fragment analysis, allele-specific real-time PCR, and circulating single-molecule amplification and resequencing technology.[71] Application of such modalities has extended to additional X-linked and autosomal recessive conditions, including spinal muscular atrophy, Gaucher disease, and Wilson disease.[72–74] cfDNA technology continues to expand, with recent studies focusing on the role of cell-free RNA and fetal-specific methylation patterns in prenatal diagnosis.[75]

FETAL BLOOD GROUP SYSTEM
Rhesus D Genotyping

The most common cause of severe hemolytic disease of the newborn is alloimmunization against the RhD red cell antigen.[76,77] Exposure of an RhD-negative woman to D antigen on the surface of fetal red blood cells activates the maternal immune system and results in alloimmunization. After maternal sensitization, all subsequent pregnancies are at risk. Neonates arising from RhD alloimmunized pregnancies may require treatment of hyperbilirubimenia and anemia.[78] Administration of anti-D immunoglobulin beginning in the 1970s has dramatically decreased the incidence of RhD alloimunization.[79] The use of cfDNA screening technology has been extended to RhD genotyping in pregnancy.[80,81]

Lo and colleagues[81] used fluorescence-based PCR to accurately assess fetal Rh status using cfDNA, thereby identifying a role for noninvasive testing in determining treatment necessity among Rh-negative women. The safety and accuracy of this approach has been established in multiple studies, allowing the routine administration of RhD anti-D prophylaxis to RhD-negative women with an RhD-positive fetus, thus avoiding unnecessary administration to women who are not at risk.[82,83]

The positive predictive value for accurate determination of fetal Rh status using cfDNA has been reported as 95% with a negative predictive value of 98% based on a large meta-analysis.[82] These findings are concordant with recent published data in the literature.[78,82–85] Application of cfDNA for Rh genotyping has emerged as the standard of care in Canada and many other European countries.[86] The Canadian RhD working group in conjunction with the Society of Obstetricians and Gynaecologists of Canada Genetics Committee summarized recent findings and cited noninvasive antenatal determination of fetal RhD genotype with cfDNA as highly accurate with sensitivities above 99% and very low false-negative rates.[87] This group and others suggest that routine treatment of all RhD-negative pregnant women with human plasma derivatives is inappropriate given no clear fetal benefit in approximately 40% of cases, particularly in the setting of maternal risk posed by Rh immune globulin exposure.[87,88] Soothill and colleagues[89] demonstrated that implementation of noninvasive fetal RhD genotyping could safely eliminate unnecessary treatment of D-negative women, thereby facilitating more appropriate allocation of resources in the setting of a current worldwide shortage of Rh immune globulin.

Despite previous concerns regarding low levels of cfDNA in early pregnancy and implications on testing sensitivity, fetal RhD genotyping has been shown to be accurate at 10 weeks' gestation.[90,91] Moise and colleagues[92] reported similar accuracy of test results across trimesters, with false-negative results (ie, a missed opportunity to prevent alloimmunization) occurring in a one of 520 cases; this mismatch was ultimately attributed to mislabeling of samples on repeat testing. These data also revealed inconclusive results in 5% to 6% of cases, attributed to the presence of the RhD pseudogene. Such early accurate testing permits targeted prophylaxis prior to 28 weeks' gestation when Rh immune globulin is typically administered, thus reducing the risk of sensitizing events prior to that time.[87] Diagnosis of an Rh-negative fetus early in pregnancy provides reassurance regarding pregnancy risk as well as reducing costs associated with potential need for serial ultrasounds and antenatal testing among pregnancies at risk of alloimmunization. Widespread use of cfDNA for RhD genotyping with selective prophylaxis awaits continued refinement of clinical and laboratory algorithms and will require ongoing interdisciplinary collaboration.[87]

Additional Blood Group Systems

Additional blood group systems have been implicated in hemolytic disease of the newborn, including the c antigen of the Rh blood group system and the K antigen of the Kell blood group system.[93] Typically blood group antigens exist as biallelic codominant systems, meaning that the fetus carries a 50% chance of acquiring the risk antigen when the father is heterozygous positive. In such scenarios, the fetus is at risk of anemia and other sequelae of severe disease. Knowledge of fetal antigen status thus allows for appropriate antenatal surveillance and management.[94] Scheffer and colleagues[84] demonstrated that noninvasive fetal blood group genotyping of antigens Rh D, c, E, and K in alloimmunized women is accurate and clinically applicable.

SUMMARY

The use of cfDNA to screen for single-gene disorders is an evolving technology, and its application is clinically limited at this time. cfDNA testing for single-gene disorders has not been well validated. Thus, patients interested in prenatal diagnosis of single-gene disorders should be offered invasive testing at this time.

cfDNA testing for the determination of fetal RhD genotype is highly accurate and considered diagnostic. The wide use of routine cfDNA determination of RhD status in the United States will likely depend on cost-effectiveness.

REFERENCES

1. Lui YYN, Chik KW, Chiu RWK, et al. Predominant hematopoietic origin of cell-free dna in plasma and serum after sex-mismatched bone marrow transplantation. Clin Chem 2002;48(3):421–7.
2. Alberry M, Maddocks D, Jones M, et al. Free fetal DNA in maternal plasma in anembryonic pregnancies: confirmation that the origin is the trophoblast. Prenat Diagn 2007;27(5):415–8.
3. Chan KCA, Zhang J, Hui ABY, et al. Size distributions of maternal and fetal DNA in maternal plasma. Clin Chem 2004;50(1):88–92.
4. Fan H, Blumenfeld Y, Chitkara U, et al. Analysis of the size distributions of fetal and maternal cell-free DNA by paired-end sequencing. Clin Chem 2010;56(8): 1279–86.
5. Ashoor G, Syngelaki A, Poon LCY, et al. Fetal fraction in maternal plasma cell-free DNA at 11-13 weeks' gestation: relation to maternal and fetal characteristics. Ultrasound Obstet Gynecol 2013;41(1):26–32.
6. ACOG. Cell- free DNA screening for fetal aneuploidy. Obstet Gynecol 2015; 126(3):e31–7.
7. Lo YM, Zhang J, Leung TN, et al. Rapid clearance of fetal DNA from maternal plasma. Am J Hum Genet 1999;64(1):218–24.

8. Herzenberg LA, Bianchi DW, Schröder J, et al. Fetal cells in the blood of pregnant women: detection and enrichment by fluorescence-activated cell sorting. Proc Natl Acad Sci U S A 1979;76(3):1453–5.
9. Lo YM, Patel P, Wainscoat JS, et al. Prenatal sex determination by DNA amplification from maternal peripheral blood. Lancet 1989;2(8676):1363–5.
10. Simpson JL, Elias S. Isolating fetal cells in maternal circulation for prenatal diagnosis. Prenat Diagn 1994;14(13):1229–42.
11. Lo YM, Lo ES, Watson N, et al. Two-way cell traffic between mother and fetus: biologic and clinical implications. Blood 1996;88(11):4390–5. Available at: http://www.ncbi.nlm.nih.gov/pubmed/8943877. Accessed November 06, 2017.
12. Lo YM, Corbetta N, Chamberlain PF, et al. Presence of fetal DNA in maternal plasma and serum. Lancet 1997;350(9076):485–7.
13. Lun FMF, Chiu RWK, Chan KCA, et al. Microfluidics digital PCR reveals a higher than expected fraction of fetal DNA in maternal plasma. Clin Chem 2008;54(10):1664–72.
14. Fan HC, Blumenfeld YJ, Chitkara U, et al. Noninvasive diagnosis of fetal aneuploidy by shotgun sequencing DNA from maternal blood. Proc Natl Acad Sci U S A 2008;105(42):16266–71.
15. Chiu RWK, Chan KCA, Gao Y, et al. Noninvasive prenatal diagnosis of fetal chromosomal aneuploidy by massively parallel genomic sequencing of DNA in maternal plasma. Proc Natl Acad Sci U S A 2008;105(51):20458–63.
16. Van den Veyver IB. Recent advances in prenatal genetic screening and testing. F1000Res 2016;5:2591.
17. Benn P, Borrell A, Crossley J, et al. Aneuploidy screening: a position statement from a committee on behalf of the Board of the International Society for Prenatal Diagnosis, January 2011. Prenat Diagn 2011;31(6):519–22.
18. Gil M, Accurti V, Santacruz B, et al. Analysis of cell-free DNA in maternal blood in screening for aneuploidies: updated meta-analysis. Ultrasound Obstet Gynecol 2017;50(3):302–14.
19. Zhou Y, Zhu Z, Gao Y, et al. Effects of maternal and fetal characteristics on cell-free fetal DNA fraction in maternal plasma. Reprod Sci 2015;22(11):1429–35.
20. Grömminger S, Erkan S, Schöck U, et al. The influence of low molecular weight heparin medication on plasma DNA in pregnant women. Prenat Diagn 2015;35(11):1155–7.
21. Norton ME, Jacobsson B, Swamy GK, et al. Cell-free DNA analysis for noninvasive examination of trisomy. N Engl J Med 2015;372(17):1589–97.
22. Livergood MC, LeChien KA, Trudell AS. Obesity and cell-free DNA "no calls": is there an optimal gestational age at time of sampling? Am J Obstet Gynecol 2017;216:413.e1-9.
23. Burns W, Koelper N, Barberio A, et al. The association between anticoagulation therapy, maternal characteristics, and a failed cfDNA test due to a low fetal fraction. Prenat Diagn 2017. https://doi.org/10.1002/pd.5152.
24. Poon LCY, Musci T, Song K, et al. Maternal plasma cell-free fetal and maternal DNA at 11-13 weeks' gestation: relation to fetal and maternal characteristics and pregnancy outcomes. Fetal Diagn Ther 2013;33(4):215–23.
25. Norton ME, Baer RJ, Wapner RJ, et al. Cell-free DNA vs sequential screening for the detection of fetal chromosomal abnormalities. Am J Obstet Gynecol 2016;214(6):727.e1-6.
26. Curnow KJ, Wilkins-Haug L, Ryan A, et al. Detection of triploid, molar, and vanishing twin pregnancies by a single-nucleotide polymorphism-based noninvasive prenatal test. Am J Obstet Gynecol 2015;212(1):79e1-9.

27. Bianchi DW, Chudova D, Sehnert AJ, et al. Noninvasive prenatal testing and incidental detection of occult maternal malignancies. JAMA 2015;314(2):162.
28. Osborne CM, Hardisty E, Devers P, et al. Discordant noninvasive prenatal testing results in a patient subsequently diagnosed with metastatic disease. Prenat Diagn 2013;33(6):609–11.
29. Brison N, Van Den Bogaert K, Dehaspe L, et al. Accuracy and clinical value of maternal incidental findings during noninvasive prenatal testing for fetal aneuploidies. Genet Med 2017;19(3):306–13.
30. Gregg AR, Skotko BG, Benkendorf JL, et al. Noninvasive prenatal screening for fetal aneuploidy, 2016 update: a position statement of the American College of Medical Genetics and Genomics. Genet Med 2016;18(10):1056–65.
31. Wax JR, Chard R, Cartin A, et al. Noninvasive prenatal testing: the importance of pretest trisomy risk and posttest predictive values. Am J Obstet Gynecol 2015; 212(4):548–9.
32. Sachs A, Blanchard L, Buchanan A, et al. Recommended pre-test counseling points for noninvasive prenatal testing using cell-free DNA: a 2015 perspective. Prenat Diagn 2015;35(10):968–71.
33. Haque IS, Lazarin GA, Kang HP, et al. Modeled fetal risk of genetic diseases identified by expanded carrier screening. JAMA 2016;316(7):734.
34. Docherty SM, Iles RK. Biomedical sciences essential laboratory medicine. Oxford (United Kingdom): John Wiley & Sons; 2012.
35. Jung A, Schuppe HC, Schill WB. Are children of older fathers at risk for genetic disorders? Andrologia 2003;35(4):191–9.
36. Friedman JM. Genetic disease in the offspring of older fathers. Obstet Gynecol 1981;57:745–9.
37. Toriello HV, Meck JM. Statement on guidance for genetic counseling in advanced paternal age. Genet Med 2008;10(6):457–60.
38. Yasuda N, Kondo K. The effect of parental age on rate of mutation for Duchenne Muscular dystrophy. Am J Med Genet 1982;13(1):91–9.
39. Tagliavacca L, Rowley G, Green P, et al. Analysis of the haemophilia A mutation in sporadic patients registered at the Royal London Hospital and their families. Haemophilia 1997;3:177–82.
40. Jackson M. Practice bulletin no. 162: prenatal diagnostic testing for genetic disorders. Obstet Gynecol 2016;127(5):e108–22.
41. Wright CF, Burton H. The use of cell-free fetal nucleic acids in maternal blood for non-invasive prenatal diagnosis. Hum Reprod Update 2009;15(1):139–51.
42. Futch T, Spinosa J, Bhatt S, et al. Initial clinical laboratory experience in noninvasive prenatal testing for fetal aneuploidy from maternal plasma DNA samples. Prenat Diagn 2013;33(6):569–74.
43. Wang J-C, Sahoo T, Schonberg S, et al. Discordant noninvasive prenatal testing and cytogenetic results: a study of 109 consecutive cases. Genet Med 2015; 17(3):234–6.
44. Verhoef TI, Hill M, Drury S, et al. Non-invasive prenatal diagnosis (NIPD) for single gene disorders: cost analysis of NIPD and invasive testing pathways. Prenat Diagn 2016;36(7):636–42.
45. Camunas-Soler J, Lee H, Hudgins L, et al. Nonivasive prenatal diagnosis of single-gene disorders using droplet digital PCR. Clin Chem 2017. [Epub ahead of print].
46. Stevenson D, Sunshine P, Benitz WE, et al. Fetal and neonatal brain injury: mechanisms, management and the risks of practice. Cambridge (United Kingdom): Cambridge University Press; 2009.

47. Krakow D, Lachman RS, Rimoin DL. Guidelines for the prenatal diagnosis of fetal skeletal dysplasias. Genet Med 2009;11(2):127–33.
48. Milunsky A, Milunsky J. Genetic disorders and the fetus: diagnosis, prevention, and treatment. Oxford (United Kingdom): John Wiley & Sons; 2015.
49. Korpi-Steiner N, Chiu RWK, Chandrasekharan S, et al. Emerging considerations for noninvasive prenatal testing. Clin Chem 2017;63(5):946–53.
50. Hill M, Twiss P, Verhoef TI, et al. Non-invasive prenatal diagnosis for cystic fibrosis: detection of paternal mutations, exploration of patient preferences and cost analysis. Prenat Diagn 2015;35(10):950–8.
51. Hill M, Compton C, Karunaratna M, et al. Client views and attitudes to non-invasive prenatal diagnosis for sickle cell disease, thalassaemia and cystic fibrosis. J Genet Couns 2014;23(6):1012–21.
52. Lewis C, Hill M, Chitty LS. Non-invasive prenatal diagnosis for single gene disorders: experience of patients. Clin Genet 2014;85(4):336–42.
53. Skirton H, Goldsmith L, Chitty LS. An easy test but a hard decision: ethical issues concerning non-invasive prenatal testing for autosomal recessive disorders. Eur J Hum Genet 2015;23(8):1004–9.
54. Pisnoli L, O'Connor A, Goldsmith L, et al. Impact of fetal or child loss on parents' perceptions of non-invasive prenatal diagnosis for autosomal recessive conditions. Midwifery 2016;34:105–10.
55. Deans Z, Clarke AJ, Newson AJ. For your interest? The ethical acceptability of using non-invasive prenatal testing to test "purely for information". Bioethics 2015;29(1):19–25.
56. Chitty LS, Mason S, Barrett AN, et al. Non-invasive prenatal diagnosis of achondroplasia and thanatophoric dysplasia: next-generation sequencing allows for a safer, more accurate, and comprehensive approach. Prenat Diagn 2015;35(7):656–62.
57. Amicucci P, Gennarelli M, Novelli G, et al. Prenatal diagnosis of myotonic dystrophy using fetal DNA obtained from maternal plasma. Clin Chem 2000;46(2):301–2.
58. González-González MC, Trujillo MJ, Rodríguez de Alba M, et al. Huntington disease-unaffected fetus diagnosed from maternal plasma using QF-PCR. Prenat Diagn 2003;23(3):232–4.
59. Meaney C, Norbury G. Noninvasive prenatal diagnosis of early onset primary dystonia I in maternal plasma. Prenat Diagn 2009;29(13):1218–21.
60. Available at: https://www.natera.com/vistara. Accessed November 06, 2017.
61. Available at: http://www.ravgen.com/single-gene-disorder-testing/. Accessed November 06, 2017.
62. Drury S, Mason S, McKay F, et al. Implementing non-invasive prenatal diagnosis (Nipd) in a national health service laboratory; From dominant to recessive disorders. Adv Exp Med Biol 2016;924:71–5.
63. Chiu RWK, Lau TK, Cheung PT, et al. Noninvasive prenatal exclusion of congenital adrenal hyperplasia by maternal plasma analysis: a feasibility study. Clin Chem 2002;48(5):778–80.
64. González-González MC, García-Hoyos M, Trujillo MJ, et al. Prenatal detection of a cystic fibrosis mutation in fetal DNA from maternal plasma. Prenat Diagn 2002;22(10):946–8.
65. Wong FCK, Lo YMD. Prenatal diagnosis innovation: genome sequencing of maternal plasma. Annu Rev Med 2016;67(1):419–32.
66. Lun FMF, Tsui NBY, Chan KCA, et al. Noninvasive prenatal diagnosis of monogenic diseases by digital size selection and relative mutation dosage on DNA in maternal plasma. Proc Natl Acad Sci U S A 2008;105(50):19920–5.

67. Barrett AN, McDonnell TCR, Chan KCA, et al. Digital PCR analysis of maternal plasma for noninvasive detection of sickle cell anemia. Clin Chem 2012;58(6): 1026–32.
68. Tsui NBY, Kadir RA, Chan KCA, et al. Noninvasive prenatal diagnosis of hemophilia by microfluidics digital PCR analysis of maternal plasma DNA. Blood 2011;117(13):3684–91.
69. Hui WWI, Jiang P, Tong YK, et al. Universal haplotype-based noninvasive prenatal testing for single gene diseases. Clin Chem 2017;63(2):513–24.
70. Hudecova I, Chiu RWK. Non-invasive prenatal diagnosis of thalassemias using maternal plasma cell free DNA. Best Pract Res Clin Obstet Gynaecol 2016;39: 63–73.
71. Allen S, Young E, Bowns B. Noninvasive prenatal diagnosis for single gene disorders. Curr Opin Obstet Gynecol 2017;29:73–9.
72. Chen M, Lu S, Lai Z, et al. Targeted sequencing of maternal plasma for haplotype-based non-invasive prenatal testing of spinal muscular atrophy. Ultrasound Obstet Gynecol 2017;49(6):799–802.
73. Zeevi DA, Altarescu G, Weinberg-Shukron A, et al. Proof-of-principle rapid noninvasive prenatal diagnosis of autosomal recessive founder mutations. J Clin Invest 2015;125(10):3757–65.
74. Lv W, Wei X, Guo R, et al. Noninvasive prenatal testing for Wilson disease by use of circulating single-molecule amplification and resequencing technology (cSMART). Clin Chem 2015;61(1):172–81.
75. Hui WWI, Chiu RWK. Noninvasive prenatal testing beyond genomic analysis: what the future holds. Curr Opin Obstet Gynecol 2016;28(2):105–10.
76. Howard H, Martlew V, McFadyen I, et al. Consequences for fetus and neonate of maternal red cell allo-immunisation. Arch Dis Child Fetal Neonatal Ed 1998;78(1): F62–6.
77. Gottvall T, Filbey D. Alloimmunization in pregnancy during the years 1992-2005 in the central west region of Sweden. Acta Obstet Gynecol Scand 2008;87(8): 843–8.
78. Tiblad E, Taune Wikman A, Ajne G, et al. Targeted routine antenatal anti-D prophylaxis in the prevention of RhD immunisation–Outcome of a new antenatal screening and prevention program. PLoS One 2013;8(8):e70984.
79. McBain RD, Crowther CA, Middleton P. Anti-D administration in pregnancy for preventing Rhesus alloimmunisation. Cochrane Database Syst Rev 2015;(9):CD000020.
80. Lo YMD, Bowell PJ, Selinger M, et al. Prenatal determination of fetal RhD status by analysis of peripheral blood of rhesus negative mothers. Lancet 1993; 341(8853):1147–8.
81. Lo YM, Hjelm NM, Fidler C, et al. Prenatal diagnosis of fetal RhD status by molecular analysis of maternal plasma. N Engl J Med 1998;339(24):1734–8.
82. Zhu Y, Zheng Y, Li L, et al. Diagnostic accuracy of non-invasive fetal RhD genotyping using cell-free fetal DNA: a meta analysis. J Matern Fetal Neonatal Med 2014;27(18):1839–44.
83. Clausen FB, Steffensen R, Christiansen M, et al. Routine noninvasive prenatal screening for fetal RHD in plasma of RhD-negative pregnant women-2years of screening experience from Denmark. Prenat Diagn 2014;34(10):1000–5.
84. Scheffer PG, Van Der Schoot CE, Page-Christiaens GCML, et al. Noninvasive fetal blood group genotyping of rhesus D, c, e and of K in alloimmunised pregnant women: evaluation of a 7-year clinical experience. BJOG 2011;118(11): 1340–8.

85. Vivanti A, Benachi A, Huchet FX, et al. Diagnostic accuracy of fetal rhesus D genotyping using cell-free fetal DNA during the first trimester of pregnancy. Am J Obstet Gynecol 2016;215(5):606.e1-5.

86. Moise KJ, Argoti PS. Management and prevention of red cell alloimmunization in pregnancy: a systematic review. Obstet Gynecol 2012;120(5):1132–9.

87. Johnson JA, MacDonald K, Clarke G, et al. No. 343-routine non-invasive prenatal prediction of fetal RHD genotype in Canada: the time is here. J Obstet Gynaecol Can 2017;39(5):366–73.

88. Kent J, Farrell A-M, Soothill P. Routine administration of Anti-D: the ethical case for offering pregnant women fetal RHDgenotyping and a review of policy and practice. BMC Pregnancy Childbirth 2014;14(1):87.

89. Soothill PW, Finning K, Latham T, et al. Use of cffDNA to avoid administration of anti-D to pregnant women when the fetus is RhD-negative: implementation in the NHS. BJOG 2015;122(12):1682–6.

90. Wikman AT, Tiblad E, Karlsson A, et al. Noninvasive single-exon fetal RHD determination in a routine screening program in early pregnancy. Obstet Gynecol 2012;120(2, Part 1):227–34.

91. Chitty LS, Finning K, Wade A, et al. Diagnostic accuracy of routine antenatal determination of fetal RHD status across gestation: population based cohort study. BMJ 2014;349:g5243.

92. Moise KJ, Gandhi M, Boring NH, et al. Circulating cell-free DNA to determine the fetal RHD status in all three trimesters of pregnancy. Obstet Gynecol 2016; 128(6):1.

93. van Wamelen DJ, Klumper FJ, de Haas M, et al. Obstetric history and antibody titer in estimating severity of Kell alloimmunization in pregnancy. Obstet Gynecol 2007;109(5):1093–8.

94. Moise KJ. Management of rhesus alloimmunization in pregnancy. Obstet Gynecol 2002;100(3):600–11.

Screening for Aneuploidy in Multiple Gestations

The Challenges and Options

Whitney Bender, MD[a], Lorraine Dugoff, MD[b],*

KEYWORDS

- Multiple gestation • Aneuploidy • Nuchal translucency • Serum screening
- Cell-free DNA • Noninvasive prenatal testing

KEY POINTS

- Although the incidence of multiple gestations has increased greatly over the last several decades, the data regarding aneuploidy screening in twins are limited.
- Screening for aneuploidy in twins using serum-based approaches is complicated because an unaffected twin may mask an affected twin. This possibility may be associated with decreased test performance compared with screening in singletons.
- Combined nuchal translucency and first-trimester serum screening with pregnancy-associated plasma protein A and beta–human chorionic gonadotropin is associated with a sensitivity and specificity of 87.4% (95% confidence interval [CI], 52.6–97.7) and 95.4% (95% CI, 94.3–96.3) in monochorionic twins and 86.2% (95% CI, 72.8–93.6) and 95.2% (95% CI, 94.2–96.0) for dichorionic twins.
- Although the data are limited, preliminary studies indicate that cell-free DNA screening may prove to be the optimal aneuploidy screening strategy for twins.
- Maternal age and nuchal translucency measurement are the only methods that can be used currently to screen for aneuploidy in higher-order multiple gestations.

INTRODUCTION

Over the past few decades, the incidence of multifetal gestations in the United States has increased markedly. Twins account for 1 in 30 live births in the United States.[1] The twinning rate increased 76% from 18.9 per 1000 births to 33.3 per 1000 births between 1980 and 2009.[1] Higher-order multiples increased by more than 400% during the same time period.[2] These trends are likely secondary to the increased use of assisted reproduction technology (ART) as well as the trend toward an older maternal age at conception.[2,3]

[a] Department of Obstetrics and Gynecology, Hospital of the University of Pennsylvania, Philadelphia, PA, USA; [b] Reproductive Genetics Division, Maternal Fetal Medicine and Reproductive Genetics University of Pennsylvania Perelman School of Medicine, 2 Silverstein Building, 3400 Spruce Street, Philadelphia, PA 19104, USA
* Corresponding author.
E-mail address: Lorraine.DugoffDr@uphs.upenn.edu

Obstet Gynecol Clin N Am 45 (2018) 41–53
https://doi.org/10.1016/j.ogc.2017.10.004
0889-8545/18/© 2017 Elsevier Inc. All rights reserved.

This article reviews the incidence of aneuploidy in twins and aneuploidy screening options for twin gestations as well as higher-order multiples. The unique challenges of aneuploidy screening in multiple gestations are also discussed.

FACTORS ASSOCIATED WITH ANEUPLOIDY IN TWIN GESTATIONS
Zygosity

Zygosity refers to the genetic makeup of the pregnancy; chorionicity, in contrast, refers to the placentation. Zygosity determines the degree of risk for chromosomal anomalies and whether or not the fetuses are concordant or discordant with regard to these risks. Monozygotic twins result from the splitting of a single fertilized ovum and, therefore, share their genetic material. Dizygotic twins result from the fertilization of 2 separate ova by 2 separate sperm, resulting in genetically distinct fetuses.

In clinical practice, the determination of zygosity is usually made from chorionicity on ultrasonography. This ultrasonography is best performed in the first trimester when the identification of the lambda or twin peak sign has been shown to be 100% accurate.[4] This sign is diagnostic of a dichorionic pregnancy. In contrast, the T sign on ultrasonography is suggestive of monochorionicity. With rare exceptions, monochorionic twins are monozygotic. From 80% to 90% of dichorionic pregnancies are dizygotic. Less than 10% arise from a single zygote that divided within 3 days postfertilization.[4–6]

Monozygotic twins

The frequency of spontaneous monozygotic twins is constant at 4 per 1000 births.[2] Monozygotic twins comprise one-third of all spontaneous twin pregnancies.[2] Because the rate of dizygotic twins increases secondary to ART, this proportion of spontaneous twin pregnancies that are monozygotic may be as much as 10 times greater.[7,8] The risk of chromosomal abnormalities in monozygotic pregnancies has historically been considered to be the same as in singleton pregnancies given the shared genetic material between the 2 fetuses. Rarely, monozygotic twins may be discordant for genetic anomalies secondary to postzygotic nondisjunction.

Dizygotic twins

The incidence of dizygotic twins varies with race, maternal age, parity, and the use of fertility treatment.[2] In dizygotic pregnancies, each fetus has an independent aneuploidy risk. Historically, it has been reported that the maternal age–related risk for each individual twin is the same as for a singleton pregnancy; therefore, the chance of 1 twin being affected for a genetic anomaly is twice that of the singleton risk. The risk of both twins being affected is the risk of the singleton squared. This risk estimation is likely oversimplified given that 10% to 20% of dichorionic twins are monozygotic.[6–8]

More recent data indicate that the incidence of aneuploidy in twins is lower than was originally reported. In a retrospective review of 77,279 twin pregnancies, including 182 with at least 1 fetus affected with Down syndrome, Sparks and colleagues[9] reported a significantly lower than expected Down syndrome incidence in women 25 to 45 years old with both monozygotic and dizygotic pregnancies. This decreased incidence of Down syndrome was most notable in monozygotic pregnancies and with increasing maternal age. The observed to expected incidence of Down syndrome per pregnancy was 33.6%, 75.2%, and 70.0% for monozygotic, dizygotic, and all twins, respectively (P<.001 for all comparisons).[9] Similar results were reported by Boyle and colleagues[10] in a retrospective study of 14.8 million births, including 427,720 multiple births. The investigators observed an adjusted relative risk of Down syndrome per fetus from multiple versus singleton pregnancies of 0.58 (95% confidence interval [CI], 0.53–0.62).[10] The lower incidence of fetal aneuploidy observed in twins may be a result of the higher rates of fetal loss associated with early spontaneous reduction of an aneuploidy twin or miscarriage of the entire twin pregnancy.[9,11]

Maternal Age

The risk of aneuploidy increases with advancing maternal age because of an increase in meiotic nondisjunction. Historically, age 35 years has been considered the lower limit for advanced maternal age. Women with singleton gestations who will be 35 years old at their due dates have a midtrimester Down syndrome risk of 1:270. The maternal age of 35 years was chosen to define advanced maternal age because the risk of Down syndrome at this age was considered to be equivalent to the risk of pregnancy loss from amniocentesis.

In monozygotic twins, advanced maternal age risk is the same as in singleton pregnancies. Because there are 2 distinct karyotypes in dizygotic twins, the risk of aneuploidy has historically been considered higher for any woman pregnant with dizygotic twins than for a woman of the same age pregnant with a singleton. Myers and colleagues[12] calculated the age-related risks for aneuploidy for twins. Their calculations took the race-related differences in dizygotic twinning into account. Using the Bayes theorem, they created charts detailing the probability of aneuploidy in at least 1 twin. The charts also assumed a fixed monozygotic twin rate of 3.5 per 1000 births. With this method, they identified 32 years as the maternal age cutoff risk for aneuploidy in twin pregnancies.[11,12]

As in singleton gestations, maternal age is an inadequate predictor of fetal aneuploidy. The sensitivity of using maternal age alone is less than 30%, with a high false-positive rate (FPR).[13] Therefore, additional aneuploidy screening methods for multifetal pregnancies are needed.

SCREENING METHODS
Ultrasonography

Nuchal translucency
Nuchal translucency (NT) is defined as the maximum thickness of the subcutaneous translucent area between the skin and the soft tissue overlying the fetal spine at the base of the neck. When measured in the sagittal plane in a fetus with a crown rump length between 38 and 84 mm, it can detect 64% to 70% of singleton fetuses with Down syndrome with an FPR of 5%.[13–15] This measurement is at maximal sensitivity when performed at 11 weeks' gestation.[14,15] In clinical practice, however, a measurement done between 11 and 14 weeks is considered valid for screening.

The advantage of NT in screening for twins is the ability to perform individual measurements on each fetus and thus generate a fetus-specific risk. The ability to obtain quality images in a multifetal pregnancy was evaluated in 2006 by Zohav and colleagues[16] in a study of 72 multiple gestations and 195 singleton gestations. There was no difference in the mean image score between multiple and singleton gestation groups.[16] Within the multiple gestation group alone, the best quality images were obtained for fetuses positioned proximal to the abdominal wall.[16] For dizygotic twins, each NT can be evaluated as a separate entity because of the distinct karyotype of each fetus. This value can then be used to assign an individual risk of aneuploidy to each fetus.

In contrast, in monozygotic twins, it becomes unclear which NT measurement to use to assign risk. Vandecruys and colleagues[17] examined 769 monochorionic twin pregnancies with NT alone at 11 weeks to 13 weeks and 6 days' gestation. Within this cohort, there were 8 cases of trisomy 21. The detection rate was 100% using the higher and average NT but 66.7% when using the smaller measurement.[17] The FPR was lowest with the use of the average NT measurement.[17] Sebire and colleagues[18] examined 448 twin pregnancies, including 95 monochorionic pregnancies, with NT at 11 to 14 weeks and reported sensitivity and FPR for trisomy 21 using combined NT and maternal age screening. Their modeled detection rate in this study was 88%.[18]

Several studies have shown an increased NT in monochorionic twins compared with dichorionic twins.[18,19] A discrepancy in the NT measurement in monochorionic twins may also be an early sign of impending twin-to-twin transfusion syndrome or selective intrauterine growth restriction.[20,21]

In addition to differences in NT caused by chorionicity, this measurement may also be affected by mode of conception. Maymon and colleagues[22] reviewed 825 twin pregnancies and found a small but significant increase in NT in ART pregnancies, particularly in vitro fertilization pregnancies. This study, however, did not find a statistically significant difference in the proportion of twins with NT values greater than the 95th percentile.[22] This difference was not found in a retrospective analysis by Hui and colleagues,[23] although his twin population was significantly smaller at only 46 pairs.

Nasal bone

The absence of a nasal bone has been associated with trisomy 21 in singletons and, when identified, may be the impetus for offering further genetic screening or a diagnostic procedure. The nasal bone marker has also been evaluated in twin pregnancies. Cleary-Goldman and colleagues[24] reported that the addition of nasal bone assessment to NT and first-trimester biomarker screening increased the Down syndrome detection rate from 79% to 89% with a 5% FPR rate in a retrospective study of 2944 twin pregnancies, including 989 dichorionic and 171 monochorionic twins.[24] It should be noted, however, that all the twins in this cohort were euploid and the detection rates were calculated using statistical modeling.[23] Therefore, although the use of the fetal nasal bone seems promising, further studies are warranted before its incorporation into routine care.

Biochemical Screening

First-trimester biochemical screening

First-trimester aneuploidy screening combines the use of NT and maternal age with the measurement of maternal serum beta–human chorionic gonadotropin (hCG) and pregnancy-associated plasma protein A (PAPP-A). In singleton pregnancies, this method has a detection rate for Down syndrome of 82% with a 5% FPR.[25] When using this technique in multiple gestations, clinicians must account for serum analyte levels that are typically double those of singleton gestations. This accounting is typically accomplished by dividing the observed multiple of the median (MoM) by the twin median to approximate a twin MoM for each analyte and plotting this number in the singleton algorithm to arrive at a risk estimate. Wald and colleagues[26,27] describe this technique and report an improved detection rate in monochorionic twins from 73% using NT and maternal age to 84% using NT, beta-hCG, PAPP-A, and maternal age for a 5% FPR.[26,27] The correction factor used may vary by center. In addition, some centers adjust for chorionicity because monochorionic twins have historically had lower levels of beta-hCG and PAPP-A than dichorionic twins.[28–30]

First-trimester biochemical screening and nuchal translucency

As with singleton pregnancies, NT seems to increase the sensitivity when added to the biochemical data. Furthermore, it is possible that an unaffected twin may mask an affected twin when analyte measurements alone are used. Therefore, first-trimester serum screening is typically combined with NT.

There are a limited number of studies reporting on first-trimester combined screening with maternal serum analytes and NT in twins. These studies are summarized in **Table 1**. Because of the limited data from affected twin pregnancies, some studies have reported theoretic performance characteristics based on modeling.[27,31] Spencer and Nicolaides[32] reported a detection rate of 75% with an FPR of 5% in a retrospective study of 206 twin pregnancies.[32] Madsen and colleagues[33] performed a retrospective study of more than 5000 twin pregnancies, including 47 trisomy 21–affected pregnancies. They showed that the addition of biochemistry to NT alone increased the detection rate for trisomy 21 from 78% to 90% in dizygotic twins with an FPR of 5.9%.[33] Similar results were reported by Chasen and colleagues[34] in a retrospective cohort study of 535 twin pregnancies including 7 fetuses in 6 dichorionic pregnancies with Down syndrome and 3 fetuses in 3 dichorionic pregnancies with trisomy 18. The use of age and NT alone identified 83% of Down syndrome and 67% of trisomy 18 pregnancies. Detection rates increased to 100% for both conditions when biochemical markers were added.[34] A retrospective study by Prats and colleagues[29] confirmed these sensitivities in a study of 447 twin pregnancies. This study additionally reported a lower FPR in monochorionic twins compared with dichorionic twins (4.4% vs 5.7%).[29] This finding is unsurprising given the identical karyotype expected in monochorionic twins; in an affected monochorionic pregnancy, the analyte values are expected to trend in the same direction. A meta-analysis including 12,794 twin fetuses with 69 cases of trisomy 21 from a total of 5 studies reported a sensitivity and specificity of 86.2% (95% CI, 72.8–93.6) and 95.2% (95% CI, 94.2–96.0) for dichorionic twins and 87.4% (95% CI, 52.6–97.7) and 95.4% (95% CI, 94.3–96.3) for monochorionic twins.[35] Of note, only 14 of the 69 cases of trisomy 21 were identified to be monochorionic twins.[35]

Pregnancies conceived with ART may have different mean analyte levels compared with spontaneous conceptions. Gjerris and colleagues[36] conducted a prospective cohort study of 1000 pregnancies and found serum PAPP-A levels to be uniformly decreased in pregnancies conceived with ART. Beta-hCG was not affected. As a result, this study found a significantly higher FPR in the ART group compared with

Table 1
Combined nuchal translucency and first-trimester biochemical screening in twin pregnancies

Study	Term Cutoff Risk	Number of Twin Pregnancies	Number of Fetuses with Trisomy 21	Detection Rate (%)	False-Positive Rate (%)
Spencer,[31] 2000	Theoretic	159	Theoretic	MZ 81.3, DZ 79.7	5.0
Wald et al,[27] 2003	Theoretic	Theoretic	Theoretic	MZ 84, DZ 70, 72 overall	5.0
Spencer & Nicolaides,[32] 2003	1:300	206	4	75 overall	6.9
Chasen et al,[34] 2007	1:300	535	7	100 overall	7.0
Prats et al,[35] 2014	1:270	447	2	MZ theoretic, DZ 100	5.7 (DZ), 4.4 (MZ)
Madsen et al,[33] 2011	1:100	5197	43	90 overall	5.9

Abbreviations: DZ, dizygotic; MZ, monozygotic.

controls.[36] Other studies have not corroborated this finding, and no studies have yet specifically examined this effect in multiple gestations. The effect of ART on first-trimester and second-trimester maternal serum analytes in twin gestations is unclear and warrants further investigation.

Second-trimester biochemical screening

Measurements of alpha fetoprotein (AFP), hCG, unconjugated estriol, and inhibin-A levels in combination with maternal age comprises second-trimester serum screening. In singleton pregnancies, the quad screen, which incorporates all 4 serum markers, has an 80% sensitivity with a 5% FPR for the detection of trisomy 21.[25] As with first-trimester screening, second-trimester analyte levels are also altered in twin pregnancies. The median unconjugated estriol value in twins is 1.6 MoM that of singleton pregnancies at the same gestational age. The MoM values are 1.84, 1.99, and 2.13 for hCG, inhibin, and AFP, respectively. These values were derived from a nested case-control study of 200 twin pregnancies and 600 singleton control pregnancies.[26,37,38] Dividing the measured result of each analyte for a woman with a twin gestation by the twin median can be used to estimate a twin MoM for each analyte. These MoM values can then be used in singleton algorithms to estimate an aneuploidy risk.

There are limited data on the performance of second-trimester screening in twins (**Table 2**). Two studies reported performance characteristics using statistical modeling.[39,40] Neveux and colleagues[39] estimated a trisomy 21 detection rate of 73% in monozygotic pregnancies and 43% in dizygotic pregnancies using a combination of maternal age and maternal serum AFP, hCG, and unconjugated estriol levels. The FPR reported in this study of 274 twin pregnancies was 5%.[39] Statistical modeling was used because no pregnancies were affected by trisomy 21. Cuckle[40] also used modeled data to predict detection rates of 41% (AFP + hCG + maternal age), 44% (AFP + hCG + unconjugated estriol + maternal age), and 47% (AFP + hCG + unconjugated estriol + inhibin-A + maternal age) of trisomy 21 in twins with a 5.0% FPR.[40]

Table 2
Second-trimester biochemical screening in twin pregnancies

Study	Term Cutoff Risk	Number of Twin Pregnancies	Number of Fetuses with Trisomy 21	Detection Rate (Screening Method) (%)	False-Positive Rate (%)
Neveux et al,[39] 1996	1:190	274	Theoretic	MC 73 DC 43 50 overall (Triple screen)	5.0
Cuckle,[40] 1998	Theoretic	Theoretic	Theoretic	41 (AFP + hCG) 44 (triple screen) 47 (quad screen)	5.0 5.0 5.0
Maymon et al,[41] 1999	1:380	60	1	100 (triple screen)	15.0
Muller et al,[42] 2003	1:250	3043	15	54.5 (AFP + hCG)	8.0
Garchet-Beaudron et al,[43] 2008	1:250	11,040	34 (20 DC twins with 1 twin affected and 7 MC twins both affected)	71 concordant 60 discordant 63 overall (AFP + hCG)	10.8

Within a cohort of 60 twin pregnancies, Maymon and colleagues[41] showed a 100% detection rate of trisomy 21 using a second-trimester triple screen (AFP, estriol, and hCG) with an FPR of 15%. Muller and colleagues[42] evaluated second-trimester AFP and hCG levels in combination with maternal age in 3043 twin gestations. There were 4 pregnancies in which both twins had Down syndrome and 7 in which 1 twin was affected. The investigators reported a detection rate of 54.5% with a 7.75% FPR using median analyte values specific to monochorionic and dichorionic twins.[42] In the largest study of second-trimester screening in twins reported to date, Garchet-Beaudron and colleagues[43] reported a mean detection rate of 63% (60% when 1 was affected and 71% when both twins were affected) and an FPR of 10.8% using a combination of maternal age, AFP, and hCG.

First and second-trimester integrated screening

To date there are no prospective studies on the use of integrated screening, involving the combination of nuchal translucency and first and second trimester maternal serum analytes, in twins. Wald and colleagues reported detection rates of 80% in all twins, 93% in monochorionic twins and 78% in dichorionic twins for a fixed false positive rate of 5% using statistical modeling.[27] There are no available data regarding the performance of the serum integrated test without nuchal translucency.

Biochemical Screening Summary

In twin pregnancies, the preferred method for Down syndrome screening is first-trimester NT combined with first-trimester biochemical screening. This method has a sensitivity between 86% and 87% at a 5% FPR. A stepwise sequential screen, which also includes a second trimester quad screen, may result in improved detection rates. Second-trimester analyte screening can be performed for patients with twin pregnancies who present for aneuploidy screening after 14 weeks' gestation. Second-trimester screening has an average detection rate of 50% to 65% at an FPR as high as 10%.

CELL-FREE DNA SCREENING

Cell-free fetal DNA was first discovered in the maternal circulation in 1997.[44] Since becoming clinically available in 2011, aneuploidy screening with this method in singletons has increased in popularity secondary to its 99% sensitivity for trisomy 21 with an FPR less than 0.02%.[45] Massive parallel sequencing is used to count cell-free DNA fragments in the plasma of pregnant women. In trisomic pregnancies, there is a small increase in the amount of a given chromosome compared with a disomic pregnancy. A fetal fraction of 4% is required by some laboratories to accurately distinguish between euploid and aneuploidy pregnancies.[46,47] These levels are usually obtained by 10 weeks of gestation in most singleton pregnancies.

There are limited studies describing the performance of cell-free DNA screening for aneuploidy in twin gestations. **Table 3** provides a summary of the studies that have been performed to date. In twin pregnancies, the total fetal fraction is generally higher secondary to the presence of additional placental tissue. Canick and colleagues[48] reported a median fetal fraction of 18.1% in twin gestations compared with 13.4% for gestational age–matched singletons. All 7 cases affected with Down syndrome, including 5 discordant and 2 concordant fetuses, were identified out of a cohort consisting of 25 twin pregnancies.[48] Bevilacqua and colleagues[49] reported cell-free DNA screen failure rates of 5.6% in 515 twin pregnancies and a 1.7% failure rate in a cohort of 1847 singleton pregnancies. They reported a median fetal fraction of 8.7% (range, 4.1%–30.0%) in twin gestations. The lower fetal fraction of the 2 fetuses was used to

Table 3
Studies of Down syndrome detection using cell-free DNA in twin gestations

Study	Gestational Age at Cell-free DNA (Mean, Range) (wk)	Number of Twin Pregnancies	Number of Fetuses with Trisomy 21	Detection Rate (95% CI) (%)	False-Positive Rate (95% CI) (%)
Canick et al,[48] 2012	Not specified (9–21)	25	7	100 (59–100)	0 (0–21)
Lau et al,[53] 2013	11.6–20.1	12	1	100 (2.5–100)	0 (0–28.5)
Huang et al,[54] 2014	19 (11–36)	189	9	100 (66.4–100)	0 (0–2.03)
del Mar Gil et al,[55] 2014	13 (12.7–13.4) for stored samples 10.6 (10–13.9) for fresh samples	275 (207 stored samples; 68 fresh samples)	12 (10 from stored samples; 2 from fresh samples)	100 in both stored and fresh samples[b]	0[b]
Bevilacqua et al,[49] 2015	13 (10–28)	515 (351 with known outcomes)	12	92[b]	0[b]
Zhang et al,[56] 2015	18.7 (9–36)	404	5	100 (47.8–100)	.50[b]
Benachi et al,[57] 2015	Not reported (first–third trimester)	7	2	100 (15.8–100)	0 (0–52.2)
Tan et al,[58] 2016	12 (11–28)	565	4	100 (39.8–100)	0 (0–0.73)
Samo et al,[50] 2016[a]	11.7 (10.4–12.9)	417	8	100 (63–100)	0 (0–0.9)
Le Conte et al,[59] 2017	16.3 (10.2–35.5)	492	3	100[b]	0.2[b]

[a] Includes some cases from the Bevilacqua and colleagues[49] study cohort.
[b] 95% CI not reported.

estimate aneuploidy risk. A higher median fetal fraction (11.3%; range, 4.0%–38.9%) was reported in the singleton cohort. Cell-free DNA screening detected 11 of the 12 trisomy 21 cases and all 5 of the trisomy 18 cases.[49] More recently, in a study that included some of the cases from the Bevilacqua and colleagues[49] study, Samo and colleagues[50] corroborated these findings of a lower median fetal fraction and higher failure rate at first sampling in twins. The screen failure rate was 9.4%. They reported a detection rate of 100% (8 out of 8) for trisomy 21% and 60% (3 out of 5) for trisomy 18 and 13 with an FPR of 0.25% in 438 twin pregnancies.[50]

As with many of the screening methods reviewed, zygosity can have a significant impact on cell-free DNA screening. Monozygotic twins, with their identical genotypes, can be considered to contribute equally to the fetal fraction. In contrast, dizygotic twins with a genetic discordance do not contribute equal amounts of genetic material in the fetal fraction. For example, a euploid twin may mask the excess genetic material contributed by a trisomic twin. This difference can be as high as 2-fold. For this reason, some studies have suggested using the lower fetal fraction of the 2 twins in the setting of dichorionic twins to estimate the risk of aneuploidy to avoid a false-negative result. This method may result in lower overall reporting rates as shown by the Bevilacqua and colleagues[49] and Samo and colleagues[50] studies.

Cell-free DNA screening using single nucleotide polymorphism–based approaches may allow the determination of zygosity, thereby avoiding the problem described earlier. Of note, this approach is not possible in cases involving donor oocytes. This approach, however, has not yet been validated in large populations.

In contrast with screening that includes the use of ultrasonography, the use of cell-free DNA screening cannot predict which twin is affected. In addition, as with many of the screening methods discussed, there is some concern that ART may result in a lower fetal fraction. Given the increased incidence of multiple gestations with ART, this may result in lower reporting rates than in spontaneously conceived twins.

Because of the challenges described earlier and the lack of validation, the American College of Obstetricians and Gynecologists, the American College of Medical Geneticists, and the National Society of Genetic Counselors do not currently recommend offering noninvasive prenatal testing to women with multiple gestations.[51]

HIGHER-ORDER MULTIPLES

In part because of the increased use of ART, higher-order multiple pregnancies, defined as triplets or greater, have also increased in frequency in the last several decades.[2] Unlike with twin gestations, an assessment of zygosity or chorionicity cannot always be reliably accomplished. Therefore, corrections for this factor in serum biomarkers are not performed.

At this time, NT measurement is the only method other than maternal age that can be used for aneuploidy screening in higher-order multiple gestations. Maymon and colleagues[52] performed a feasibility study of 24 pregnant women carrying 79 fetuses and compared their NT measurements with singleton controls. NT measurement distributions among the multiples were similar to those of their gestational age–matched controls.[52]

SUMMARY

The incidence of multiple gestations has increased dramatically in the last several decades and is likely to continue to increase as average maternal age and the use of ART increase. The risk of aneuploidy varies based on age and zygosity. At present, the use of NT, which can generate a fetus-specific risk, in combination with first-trimester maternal serum analytes seems to be the most reliable screening approach in twins. The measurement of NT combined with maternal age is the only option available for genetic screening in higher-order multiples. Although the available data regarding cell-free DNA screening in twins are promising, additional studies are required to better define the performance characteristics.

REFERENCES

1. Martin JA, Hamilton BE, Osterman MLK. Three decades of twin births in the United States, 1980–2009. NCHS Data Brief 2012;80:1–8.
2. American College of Obstetricians and Gynecologists. ACOG practice bulletin no.144: multifetal gestations: twin, triplet, and higher-order multifetal pregnancies. Obstet Gynecol 2014;123(5):1118–32.
3. Blondel B, Kaminski M. Trends in the occurrence, determinants, and consequences of multiple births. Semin Perinatol 2002;26:239–49.
4. Sepulveda W, Sebire NJ, Hughes K, et al. Evolution of the lambda or twin-chorionic peak sign in dichorionic twin pregnancies. Obstet Gynecol 1997;89:439–41.
5. Machin GA. Why is it important to diagnose chorionicity and how do we do it? Best Pract Res Clin Obstet Gynaecol 2004;18:515–30.
6. Gagnon A, Audibert F. Prenatal screening and diagnosis of aneuploidy in multiple pregnancies. Best Pract Res Clin Obstet Gynaecol 2014;28:285–94.
7. Jenkins TM, Wapner RJ. The challenge of prenatal diagnosis in twin pregnancies. Curr Opin Obstet Gynecol 2000;12:87–92.
8. Cleary-Goldman J, D'Alton ME, Berkowitz RL. Prenatal diagnosis and multiple pregnancy. Semin Perinatol 2005;29:312–20.
9. Sparks TN, Norton ME, Flessel M, et al. Observed rate of down syndrome in twin pregnancies. Obstet Gynecol 2016;128(5):1127–33.
10. Boyle B, Morris JK, McConkey R, et al. Prevalence and risk of Down syndrome in monozygotic and dizygotic multiple pregnancies in Europe: implications for prenatal screening. BJOG 2014;121(7):809–19.
11. Rodis FJ, Egan JFX, Craffy A, et al. Calculated risks of chromosomal abnormalities in twin gestations. Obstet Gynecol 1990;76:1037.
12. Myers C, Adam R, Dungan J, et al. Aneuploidy in twin gestations: when is maternal age advanced? Obstet Gynecol 1997;89:248.
13. Odibo AO, Lawrence-Clearly K, Macones GA. Screening for aneuploidy in twins and higher-order multiples: is first-trimester nuchal translucency the solution? Obstet Gynecol Surv 2002;58:609–14.
14. Malone FD, Canick JA, Ball RH, et al. First-trimester or second-trimester screening, or both, for Down's syndrome. N Engl J Med 2005;353(19):2001–11.
15. Simpson LL. Ultrasound in twins: dichorionic and monochorionic. Semin Perinatol 2013;37:348–58.
16. Zohav E, Segal O, Rabinson J, et al. Quality of nuchal translucency measurements in multifetal pregnancies. J Matern Fetal Neonatal Med 2006;19(10):663–6.
17. Vandecruys H, Faiola S, Auer M, et al. Screening for trisomy 21 in monochorionic twins by measurement of fetal nuchal translucency thickness. Ultrasound Obstet Gynecol 2005;25:551–3.
18. Sebire NJ, Snijders RJ, Hughes K, et al. Screening for trisomy 21 in twin pregnancies by maternal age and fetal nuchal translucency thickness at 10-14 weeks of gestation. Br J Obstet Gynaecol 1996;103(10):999–1003.

19. Cheng PJ, Huang SY, Shaw SW, et al. Difference in nuchal translucency between monozygotic and dizygotic spontaneously conceived twins. Prenat Diagn 2010; 30:247–50.

20. Bora SA, Bourne T, Bottomley C, et al. Twin growth discrepancy in early pregnancy. Ultrasound Obstet Gynecol 2009;34:38–42.

21. Sebire NJ, D'Ercole C, Hughes K, et al. Increased nuchal translucency thickness at 10-14 weeks of gestation as a predictor of severe twin-to-twin transfusion syndrome. Ultrasound Obstet Gynecol 1997;10:86–9.

22. Maymon R, Cuckle H, Svirsky R, et al. Nuchal translucency in twins according to mode of assisted conception and chorionicity. Ultrasound Obstet Gynecol 2014; 44:38–43.

23. Hui PW, Tang MH, Ng EH, et al. Nuchal translucency in dichorionic twins conceived after assisted reproduction. Prenat Diagn 2006;26(6):510–3.

24. Cleary-Goldman J, Rebarber A, Krantz D, et al. First trimester screening with nasal bone in twins. Am J Obstet Gynecol 2008;199:283.e1-3.

25. American College of Obstetricians and Gynecologists. ACOG practice bulletin no 77: screening for fetal chromosomal abnormalities. Obstet Gynecol 2007;109: 217–27.

26. Wald N, Cuckle H, Wu T. Maternal serum un-conjugated estriol and human chorionic gonadotropin levels in twin pregnancies: implications for screening for Down's syndrome. Br J Obstet Gynaecol 1991;98:905–8.

27. Wald N, Rish S, Hacksaw AK. Combining nuchal translucency and serum markers in prenatal screening for down syndrome in twin pregnancy. Prenat Diagn 2003;23:588–92.

28. Spencer K, Kagan KO, Nicolaides KH. Screening for trisomy 21 in twin pregnancies in the first trimester: an update of the impact of chorionicity on maternal serum markers. Prenat Diagn 2008;28:49–52.

29. Prats P, Rodriguez I, Comas C, et al. First trimester risk assessment for trisomy 21 in twin pregnancies combining nuchal translucency and first trimester biochemical markers. Prenat Diagn 2012;32:927–32.

30. Vink J, Wapner R, D'Alton ME. Prenatal diagnosis in twin gestation. Semin Perinatol 2012;36:169–74.

31. Spencer K. Screening for trisomy 21 in twin pregnancies in the first trimester using free beta-hCG and PAPP-A, combined with fetal nuchal translucency thickness. Prenat Diagn 2000;20(2):91–5.

32. Spencer K, Nicolaides KH. Screening for trisomy 21 in twins using first trimester ultrasound and maternal serum biochemistry in a one-stop clinic: a review of three years of experience. BJOG 2003;110:276–80.

33. Madsen HN, Ball S, Wright D, et al. A reassessment of biochemical marker distributions in trisomy 21 affected and unaffected twin pregnancies in the first trimester. Ultrasound Obstet Gynecol 2011;37:38–47.

34. Chasen ST, Perni SC, Kalish RB, et al. First trimester risk assessment for trisomies T21 and 18 in twin pregnancy. Am J Obstet Gynecol 2007;197:374.e1-3.

35. Prats P, Rodriguez I, Comas C, et al. Systematic review of screening for trisomy 21 in twin pregnancies in first trimester combining nuchal translucency and biochemical markers: a meta-analysis. Prenat Diagn 2014;34:1077–83.

36. Gjerris AC, Loft A, Pinborg A, et al. First trimester screening markers are altered in pregnancies conceived after IVF/ICSI. Ultrasound Obstet Gynecol 2009;33:8–17.

37. Wald NJ, Densem JW. Maternal serum free alpha-human chorionic gonadotropin levels in twin pregnancies: implications for screening for Down's syndrome. Prenat Diagn 1994;14(8):717–9.

38. Watt HC, Wald NJ, George L. Maternal serum inhibin-A levels in twin pregnancies: implications for screening for Down's syndrome. Prenat Diagn 1996;16(10):927–9.
39. Neveux LM, Palomaki GE, Knight GJ, et al. Multiple marker screening for Down syndrome in twin pregnancies. Prenat Diagn 1996;16:29–34.
40. Cuckle H. Down's syndrome screening in twins. J Med Screen 1998;5:3–4.
41. Maymon R, Dreazen E, Rozinsky S, et al. Comparison of nuchal translucency measurement and second-trimester triple serum screening in twin versus singleton pregnancies. Prenat Diagn 1999;19(8):727–31.
42. Muller F, Dreux S, Dupoizat H. Second trimester Down syndrome maternal serum screening in twin pregnancies: impact of chorionicity. Prenat Diagn 2003;23(4):331–5.
43. Garchet-Beaudron A, Dreux S, Leporrier N, et al. Second trimester Down syndrome maternal serum marker screening: a prospective study of 11040 twin pregnancies. Prenat Diagn 2008;28(12):1105–9.
44. Lo YM, Corbetta N, Chamberlain PF, et al. Presence of fetal DNA in maternal plasma and serum. Lancet 1997;350:485–7.
45. Mackie FL, Hemming K, Allen S, et al. The accuracy of cell-free fetal DNA-based non-invasive prenatal testing in singleton pregnancies: a systematic review and bivariate meta-analysis. BJOG 2017;124:32–46.
46. Palomaki GE, Kloza EM, Lambert-Messerlian GM, et al. DNA sequencing of maternal plasma to detect Down syndrome: an international clinical validation study. Genet Med 2011;13:913–20.
47. Norton ME, Brar H, Weiss J, et al. Non-invasive chromosomal evaluation study: results of a multicenter prospective study for detection of fetal trisomy 21 and trisomy 18. Am J Obstet Gynecol 2012;207:137.e1-8.
48. Canick JA, Kloza EM, Lembert-Messerlian GM, et al. DNA sequencing of maternal plasma to identify Down syndrome and other trisomies in multiple gestations. Prenat Diagn 2012;32:730–4.
49. Bevilacqua E, Bil MM, Nicolaides KH, et al. Performance of screening for aneuploidies by cell-free DNA analysis of maternal blood in twin pregnancies. Ultrasound Obstet Gynecol 2015;45(1):61–6.
50. Samo L, Revello R, Hanson E, et al. Prospective first-trimester screening for trisomies by cell-free DNA testing of maternal blood in twin pregnancy. Ultrasound Obstet Gynecol 2016;47(6):705–11.
51. American College of Obstetricians and Gynecologists. Noninvasive prenatal testing for fetal aneuploidy. Committee opinion no. 545. Obstet Gynecol 2012; 120:1532–4.
52. Maymon R, Dreazen E, Tovbin Y, et al. The feasibility of nuchal translucency measurement in higher order multiple gestations achieved by assisted reproduction. Hum Reprod 1999;14:2102–5.
53. Lau TK, Fuman J, Chan MK, et al. Non-invasive prenatal screening of fetal Down syndrome by maternal plasma DNA sequencing in twin pregnancies. J Matern Fetal Neonatal Med 2013;26:434–7.
54. Huang X, Zheng J, Chen M, et al. Noninvasive prenatal testing of trisomies 21 and 18 by massively parallel sequencing of maternal plasma DNA in twin pregnancies. Prenat Diagn 2014;34(4):335–40.
55. Del Mar Gil M, Quezada MS, Breant B, et al. Cell-free DNA analysis for trisomy risk assessment in first trimester twin pregnancies. Fetal Diagn Ther 2014;35:204–11.
56. Zhang H, Gao Y, Jiang F, et al. Non-invasive prenatal testing for trisomies 21, 18, and 13: clinical experience from 146, 958 pregnancies. Ultrasound Obstet Gynecol 2015;45(5):530–8.

57. Benachi A, Letourneau A, Kleinfinger P, et al. Cell-free DNA analysis in maternal plasma in cases of fetal abnormalities detected on ultrasound examination. Obstet Gynecol 2015;125(6):1330–7.
58. Tan Y, Gao Y, Ge L, et al. Noninvasive prenatal testing (NIPT) in twin pregnancies with treatment of assisted reproductive techniques (ART) in a single center. Prenat Diagn 2016;36(7):672–9.
59. Le Conte G, Letourneau A, Jani J, et al. Cell-free DNA analysis in maternal plasma as a screening test for trisomy 21, 18 and 13 in twin pregnancies. Ultrasound Obstet Gynecol 2017. [Epub ahead of print].

The Use of Chromosomal Microarray Analysis in Prenatal Diagnosis

Melissa Stosic, MS[a], Brynn Levy, MSc (Med), PhD[b],
Ronald Wapner, MD[a],*

KEYWORDS

- Prenatal array • Chromosomal microarray • Prenatal diagnosis • Array CGH

KEY POINTS

- Copy number variants of well-defined clinical significance not identifiable by standard karyotype are not associated with maternal age and occur in 1% to 1.7% of routine pregnancies and in 6% of pregnancies with ultrasound anomalies.
- Chromosomal microarray analysis (CMA) is the currently recommended primary test for cytogenetic analysis of all pregnancies undergoing invasive testing after identification of a fetal ultrasound abnormality.
- All women having invasive testing for routine indications such as maternal age, anxiety, and abnormal serum screening can be offered microarray as an option.
- For any patient pursuing CMA, pretest counseling is imperative for them to understand the benefits and limitations, and to make an appropriate decision regarding testing.
- For patients with abnormal CMA results, including those with variants of uncertain significance, posttest counseling should be in-depth and be conducted by a practitioner with full knowledge of the implications of the result, such as a genetic counselor or clinical geneticist.

INTRODUCTION

Prenatal cytogenetic diagnosis has expanded over the past several years from karyotype and fluorescence in situ hybridization to chromosomal microarray analysis (CMA). This evolution to CMA occurred simultaneously with the realization that many childhood anomalies and developmental disorders are secondary to small deletions and duplications previously unrecognized by standard karyotype. Many of

Financial Disclosures: Ronald Wapner, MD, is funded in part by a NICHD grant (1U01HD055651) on prenatal microarray and Melissa Stosic, MS, has been supported in part by the same grant.
[a] Department of Obstetrics and Gynecology, Columbia University Medical Center, 622 West 168th Street, New York, NY 10032, USA; [b] Department of Pathology and Cell Biology, Columbia University Medical Center, 622 West 168th Street, New York, NY 10032, USA
* Corresponding author.
E-mail address: rw2191@cumc.columbia.edu

these explained the causes of previously described syndromes, whereas others were identified as the previously unsuspected cause of neurocognitive disabilities. **Table 1** lists many of the common microdeletion syndromes and copy number variants (CNVs) associated with neurocognitive disorders such as autism and intellectual disability.

In pediatrics, CMA has rapidly become a mainstay for diagnosis in children with developmental delay or intellectual disability, autism spectrum disorders, and/or multiple congenital anomalies. It is now recognized as the first-tier test (superseding karyotype) for these disorders.[1] Approximately 15% of such cases will demonstrate a causative CNV despite a normal karyotype.[2]

In 2013, the American Congress of Obstetricians and Gynecologists (ACOG) along with the Society for Maternal Fetal Medicine (SMFM) released recommendations that CMA replace or supplement karyotype for prenatal evaluation of fetuses with major structural anomalies. They also suggested that either karyotype or CMA is appropriate for women with structurally normal fetuses undergoing diagnostic prenatal testing. In addition, they clarified that microdeletions or duplications are not associated with advanced maternal age (AMA) and, therefore, CMA should not be restricted to women older than 35 years of age.[3] This aligns with the ACOG statement in place since 2007, which states that all pregnant women should be offered the option of diagnostic testing regardless of maternal age.[4,5]

With the increasingly better performance of noninvasive screening for pregnancies with a common chromosomal abnormality (trisomies 21, 18, and 13, and sex chromosome abnormalities) the rates of invasive diagnostic procedures have declined. However, simultaneously, the introduction of CMA has made available diagnosis of an increased spectrum of cytogenetic disorders; many with phenotypes as severe as those of the common aneuploides.[6] Given the options now available to pregnant women, an understanding of the scope and accuracy of CMA becomes an important part of the broader picture. This article focuses on an overview of CMA, including common microdeletion and duplication syndromes, the different methodologies available, how it fits into prenatal care, and the critical counseling components.

CHROMOSOMAL MICROARRAY TECHNOLOGY

Historically, karyotype has been the primary approach to analysis on chorionic villus and amniocentesis samples. With a resolution of 7 to 10 Megabases (Mb) or million base pairs, it is able to detect whole chromosome aneuploidy and structural aberrations such as large deletions or duplications. However, the limitations of light microscopy prevent the diagnosis of submicroscopic changes such as microdeletions and duplications less than 7 to 10 Mb; some being as small as tens to hundreds of thousands of base pairs (kilobases). Identification of these requires testing using molecular cytogenomic techniques such as CMA. There are 2 main types of CMA performed currently: oligonucleotide and single nucleotide polymorphism (SNP) microarray.

Oligonucleotide Array Comparative Genomic Hybridization Versus Single Nucleotide Polymorphism Microarray

Array comparative genomic hybridization (aCGH) technology directly compares short DNA fragments from a patient sample to a reference sample to determine if there is a shortage (deletion) or excess (duplication) of patient DNA relative to reference DNA at specific loci (**Fig. 1**). The control element on the array is generally a synthetic short stretch ($\sim$25–35 base pairs) of DNA of known sequence and chromosomal location, called an oligonucleotide.

Table 1
Common microdeletion and duplication syndromes and frequency of occurrence

Condition, Genomic Location	Incidence	Major Phenotypic Features
16p11.2 duplication	1/1900	Normal to DD, ASD, ADHD, microcephaly, psychiatric conditions
16p11.2 deletion	1/2300	ID or DD, ASD, ADHD, macrocephaly, psychiatric conditions
16p13.11 deletion	1/2300	ID or DD, seizures, schizophrenia
1q21.1 duplication	1/3300	Normal to motor skill and articulation difficulty, ID or DD, ASD, ADHD, scoliosis, abnormal gait, macrocephaly, short stature, psychiatric conditions (schizophrenia, anxiety, depression), CHD (especially tetralogy of Fallot)
22q11.2 deletion syndrome (DiGeorge, velocardiofacial syndrome)	1/4000	CHD (most commonly conotruncal), palate abnormalities, characteristic facies, ID or DD, immune deficiency, hypocalcemia, psychiatric conditions in early adulthood (schizophrenia, depression, bipolar disorder)
22q11.2 duplication	1/4000	Normal to ID or DD, growth retardation, hypotonia
1p36 deletion syndrome	1/5000	ID or DD, hypotonia, seizures, structural brain abnormalities, CHD, vision and hearing issues, skeletal anomalies, characteristic facies
Charcot-Marie-Tooth type 1A; 17p12 duplication	1/5000–1/10,000	Slowly progressive neuropathy causing distal muscle weakness and atrophy, sensory loss, and slow nerve conduction velocity, first noticeable in the first or second decade
X-linked ichthyosis; Xp22.31 deletion	1/6000	ID or DD, ichthyosis, Kallman syndrome, short stature, ocular albinism
Williams syndrome; 7q11.23 deletion	1/7500	ID or DD, cardiovascular disease, characteristic facies, connective tissue abnormalities, specific personality, growth anomalies, endocrine abnormalities
7q11.23 duplication	1/7500	DD, normal to ID intellectually, speech problems, hypotonia, problems with movement and walking, behavioral abnormalities, seizures, aortic enlargement
Prader-Willi syndrome; 15q11.2 paternal deletion	1/10,000	ID or DD, hypotonia and feeding difficulties in infancy, excessive eating, obesity, behavioral difficulties, hypogonadism, short stature
Angelman syndrome; 15q11.2 maternal deletion	1/12,000	ID or DD, severe speech impairment, gait ataxia, inappropriate happy affect, microcephaly, seizures
17q12 deletion	1/14,500	Kidney or urinary abnormalities, diabetes, ID or DD, ASD, psychiatric conditions
Sotos syndrome; 5q35 deletion	1/15,000	ID or DD, overgrowth, characteristic facies

(continued on next page)

Table 1
(*continued*)

Condition, Genomic Location	Incidence	Major Phenotypic Features
Smith-Magenis syndrome; 17p11.2 deletion	1/15,000–1/25,000	ID or DD, characteristic facies, sleep disturbances, behavioral issues including self-injury and self-hugging and aggression, characteristic facies, reduced sensitivity to pain and temperature
Cri-du-chat; 5p15 deletion	1/15,000–1/50,000	High-pitched cry, microcephaly, hypotonia, characteristic facies, ID or DD, CHD
Koolen de Vries; 17q21 deletion	1/16,000	ID or DD, sociable personality, hypotonia, seizures, distinct facial features, CHD, kidney anomalies, foot deformities
Potocki-Lupski syndrome; 17p11.2 duplication	1/20,000	ID or DD, ASD, hypotonia, CHD

Abbreviations: ADHD, attention deficit hyperactivity disorder; ASD, autism spectrum disorder; CHD, congenital heart defect; DD, developmental delay; ID, intellectual disability.

SNP microarrays, on the other hand, do not use a comparative reference sample, but rather determine the genotype of the patient at specific areas of the genome that are highly polymorphic (different) between individuals. These differences are termed SNPs. By determining the genotype at millions of polymorphic locations, absent or duplicated stretches of DNA can be recognized (**Fig. 2**). The advantage of the SNP array is that it can also identify long contiguous stretches of homozygosity (LCSH), which could indicate uniparental disomy (UPD), in which a child has inherited 2 copies of a chromosome from 1 parent rather than 1 copy from each parent, or consanguinity, and can be responsible for an underlying genetic condition if it involves one of the imprinted chromosomes. LCSH could also increase the risk of homozygosity for a recessive condition in one of those regions. Unlike aCGH, which compares the relative amounts of DNA from various areas of the genome and hence could not identify triploidy in which all areas are simultaneously increased, SNP arrays can identify triploidy.

Targeted Versus Whole Genome Arrays

The ability of an array to identify CNVs depends on the coverage of the individual array platform. Some arrays are designed to only target specific critical regions of the genome proven to be associated with known genetic conditions. Whole genome arrays include dense targeted coverage over known critical regions to identify even small CNVs in these regions. In addition, these have broader coverage across the rest of the genome (referred to as the backbone) to detect slightly larger deletions and duplications in any region. The backbone coverage differs by laboratory and platform but prenatally is generally .5 to 1 Mb. However, the targeted approach has been proven to have only a limited impact on reducing identification of benign variants or variants of uncertain significance.[7]

CHROMOSOMAL MICROARRAY ANALYSIS REPORTING

American College of Medical Genetics and Genomics (ACMG), in collaboration with the Association for Molecular Pathology, has published guidelines for the interpretation of variants and suggested a 5-tier system of reporting.[8] With this system, variants

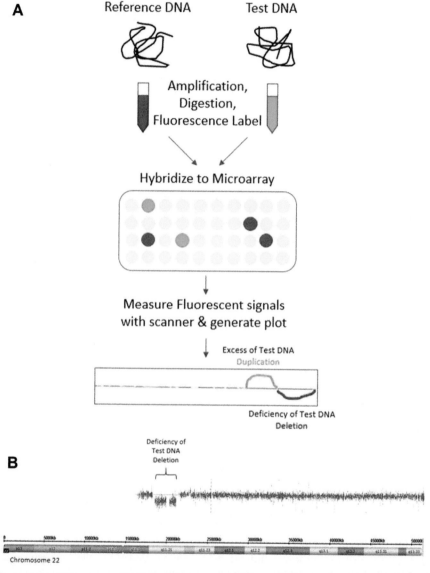

Fig. 1. Array CGH process. (*A*) The aCGH process, which results in determination of the ratio of reference to test DNA at each oligonucleotide on the array. This ratio shows if there is an excess or deficiency of test DNA, and is used to identify imbalances such as whole chromosome aneuploidy or microdeletions or duplications. Red signifies a deletion of test DNA and green signifies a duplication of test DNA. (*B*) The actual generated image of the copy number plot from an aCGH platform on a case with approximately 3 Mb deletion of 22q11.2.

are interpreted as pathogenic, likely pathogenic, uncertain significance, likely benign, or benign. Each report should include the following[9]:

- Cytogenetic location (chromosome number and band)
- Whether it is a loss or gain of copy number and mechanism, if known

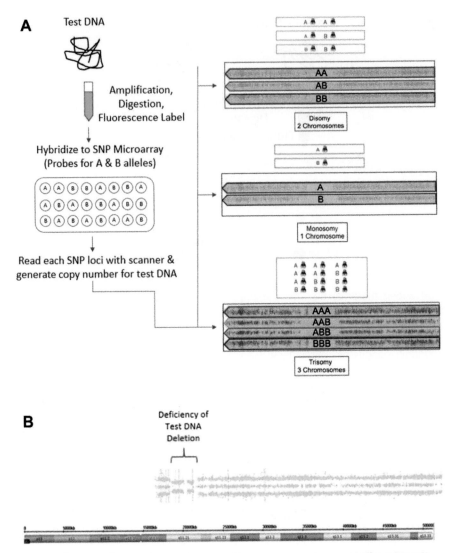

Fig. 2. (*A*) The SNP array process, which results in determination of the allele at each loci on the array. The alleles are then used to determine copy number to identify imbalances such as whole chromosome aneuploidy or microdeletions or duplications. (*B*) The actual generated image from an SNP array platform.

- CNV size and coordinates with genome build (ie, hg19)
- Statement of significance as previously defined (including evidence and references)
- Genes involved (if a known syndrome, those related to that condition; If uncertain CNV, all the reference sequence (RefSeq) genes)
- Recommendations for appropriate clinical follow-up.

It is not unusual for interpretation of the clinical significance of a CNV to be complex; especially if it is a variant of uncertain significance. In these cases, consultation of the laboratory with a clinical geneticist and discussion with the ordering clinician can add important insight in addition to the written report.

THE ROLE OF CHROMOSOMAL MICROARRAY ANALYSIS IN PRENATAL DIAGNOSIS
Chromosomal Microarray Analysis Versus Karyotype

In addition to the obvious broader identification of anomalies via detection of microdeletion and duplication syndromes, according to the ACMG, the advantages of CMA compared with karyotype are[10]

- Broader range of tissue types can be analyzed and no tissue culture is necessary (CMA can be performed on DNA extracted from uncultured villi, amniotic fluid, and fetal tissue and blood, including stored samples and paraffin blocks)
- Identification of findings that are cryptic by standard karyotype
- Platforms are customizable to focus on areas of interest
- Better delineation of findings identified on karyotype
- Objective rather than subjective evaluation
- Detection of LCSH (including UPD) with SNP-based platforms
- Resulting data are compatible with genome browsers and databases.

The disadvantages are

- Inability to identify balanced rearrangements (will be seen by karyotype but does not have clinical significance for the present pregnancy)
- Potential to miss low-level mosaicism (although karyotypes can also miss low-level mosaicism)
- Lack of information about the mechanism of the CNV (karyotypes will provide this information in most cases; eg, unbalanced translocation, marker chromosome)
- Tetraploidy (SNP) and/or triploidy (aCGH) may be missed (will be identified by karyotype)
- CNVs outside of the platform coverage or minimum reporting size are missed (these will also be missed by karyotype)
- Point mutations, gene expression, and methylation anomalies are not identified (these are also not identifiable by karyotype)
- Negative array does not 100% rule out a condition due to individual mutations, small size, and other genomic causes.

The SMFM recommends that all women who are undergoing diagnostic testing be given information about both karyotype and CMA, and have the option of choosing which to have.[11] Because there are advantages to both approaches, some laboratories have adopted the approach of doing both analyses. In this case, CMA is used as the primary diagnostic tool because of its ability to expand the clinically relevant diagnostic results, and karyotype is used to avoid missing balanced changes and to help in the evaluation of the underlying mechanism, which may have important implications for future pregnancies. Karyotype may also be of benefit in identifying low levels of mosaicism; however, it should be remembered that the standard approach to karyotyping, in which 15 cells are counted, will only detect 15% mosaicism at 90% confidence, 19% mosaicism at 95% confidence, or 27% mosaicism and 99% confidence.[12] In these cases cell culture provides the ability to obtain and count more cells.

Chromosomal Microarray Analysis as Routine Testing

The initial clinical value of CMA for routine prenatal evaluation was published in the New England Journal of Medicine (NEJM) and blindly compared karyotype results to CMA. The study demonstrated that, in pregnancies with a normal karyotype sampled by chorionic villus sampling (CVS) or amniocentesis and with no anomalies on ultrasound (ie, sampled for AMA, abnormal maternal serum screening, or anxiety) clinically relevant CNVs were seen in 1.7% of cases.[6] A metaanalysis was recently conducted that included the 10 largest studies of CMA for prenatal evaluation (10,614 fetuses). In 0.84% (95% CI 0.55–1.30) of fetuses a submicroscopic pathogenic aberration was detected prenatally. The onset or penetrance of the submicroscopic findings was studied in 10,314 fetuses from 8 papers that presented aberrant cases with all necessary details. The pooled estimates indicated that in 0.37% (95% CI 0.27–0.52) an early-onset syndromic disorder was detected, in 0.30% (95% CI 0.14–0.67) a susceptibility CNV was found, and in 0.11% (95% CI 0.05–0.21) cases of late onset diseases were reported. The prevalence of early-onset syndromic disorders due to a submicroscopic aberration was calculated to be 1 per 270. When the risk for submicroscopic aberrations was added to the individual risk for microscopic chromosome aberrations, all pregnant women have a risk higher than 1 per 180 for a relevant chromosome aberration and pregnant women younger than 36 years old have a higher risk for submicroscopic pathogenic aberrations than for Down syndrome.[13]

As seen in **Table 2** the frequency of incremental results varies between studies. This variation is likely due to local definitions of the pathogenicity of specific results, which has changed over time. In the initial NEJM article, the incidence of variants of uncertain significance as reported to patients was 2.5%. Over the next 7 years, rereview of the interpretation of the CNVs reduced this to 0.9% based on new literature.[14]

In a large systematic review, 2.4% of cases overall (including those with and without structural abnormalities) had a clinically significant finding on CMA that was not identified by karyotype. This decreased to 1% in the population referred for AMA, abnormal maternal serum screening, and anxiety.[19] Overall, the incremental yield of microarray over karyotype in fetuses without anomalies has been shown to be 1% to 2%.

Table 2
Reports evaluating the incremental yield of chromosomal microarray analysis compared with karyotype in fetuses without anomalies

Article Author, Year	Number of Cases	Incremental Yield Over Karyotype[a]	Incidence of VOUS
Wapner et al,[6] 2012, Wapner,[14] 2015	2695[b]	1.7%	0.9% (2.5% reported during study)
Van Opstal et al,[15] 2015	1330[c]	2.0%	0.5% reported as likely pathogenic
Bornstein et al,[16] 2017	931[d]	0.4%	1.5%
Shaffer et al,[17] 2012	518[e]	.96%	2.7% (0.39% if only de novo considered)
Scott et al,[18] 2013	1049[f]	1.2%	0.3%

[a] Including variants of uncertain significance (VOUS) that are likely pathogenic.
[b] Excludes 372 marked as other.
[c] Of this 2.0%, 0.1% were causative, 1.4% were susceptibility loci, and 0.6% were unexpected diagnoses not explaining the phenotypes, such as late-onset conditions.
[d] Includes referrals for AMA and parental desire.
[e] The 518 were referred for AMA, maternal anxiety, or abnormal serum screening.
[f] Indications include AMA, abnormal serum screening, and anxiety.

Chromosomal Microarray Analysis in Fetuses with Ultrasound Anomalies

There are well-known associations between CNVs and specific fetal anomalies; for example, cardiac defects and deletions of 22q11.2, leading to DiGeorge syndrome, or lissencephaly and Miller-Dieker syndrome (17p13.3 deletion). In addition, UPD, which can be identified by CMA (eg, Beckwith-Wiedmann syndrome and Russell-Silver syndrome) can present with ultrasound-identifiable anomalies.[20,21] Because CMA has ability to better define the underlying cause of a fetal structural anomaly, leading to improved counseling, the ACOG recommends CMA be performed on patients undergoing invasive testing for 1 or more structural ultrasound anomalies.[11,22] In addition, because CMA does not require tissue culture, which is frequently difficult or impossible on stillborn tissue, CMA is also recommended in these cases.[23]

Several large-scale studies evaluating the incremental yield of CMA in fetuses with ultrasound anomalies have been published. In a 2012 study, clinically significant findings were identified in 6% of fetuses with a normal karyotype and an ultrasound anomaly.[6] Srebniak and colleagues[24] used SNP arrays to test 1033 fetuses with ultrasound anomalies and found 57 (5.5%) had a pathogenic abnormality not visible on karyotype. In a large study of 5000 cases of which 2462 had ultrasound anomalies, the additional yield of microarray over karyotype was 6.6% in the anomalous cohort.[17] A metaanalysis by Hillman and colleagues[25] found that CMA identified an additional 7% to 10% over karyotype in pregnancies with structural abnormalities. A second metaanalysis found 7.0% incremental yield of CMA in pregnancies with ultrasound anomalies.[19] Overall, the literature clearly demonstrates that CMA will provide additional information over karyotype in about 6% to 7% of pregnancies when the fetus has an anomaly.

The likelihood of CMA revealing a clinically significant finding in a patient with an ultrasound anomaly also depends on the system involved and whether single or multiple anomalies are seen. The abnormalities most commonly associated with abnormal CMA results are cardiac, skeletal, urogenital, renal, and central nervous system.[26–29] Patients with structural anomalies in more than 1 system have a 13% frequency of a significant or potentially significant CNV versus 5.1% in those with an isolated abnormality.[30]

Comparison of Diagnostic Testing Versus Screening for Prenatal Surveillance

As screening performance has improved, many women who previously might have considered CVS or amniocentesis with CMA analysis are now choosing noninvasive screening by nuchal translucency and biochemistry or by cell-free DNA screening that, in most cases, is limited to the common chromosome abnormalities. In some women, this choice is easy because they are attempting to avoid any risks associated with a diagnostic procedure and are willing to sacrifice the additional information CMA offers to accomplish this. However, many women are unaware of the incremental information that CMA might provide.

When discussing screening for genetic disorders, Down syndrome is commonly thought of as the main focus. This is partially historical because for almost half a century this was true because technology to identify other cytogenetic disorders, such as CNVs, did not exist. In addition, many women incorrectly interpret Down syndrome as meaning any child with intellectual disability and are not aware that it specifically refers to trisomy 21, meaning they may believe that a noninvasive screening test for Down syndrome has a much broader testing capability. For these reasons, it is critical that patients understand the benefits and limitations of both approaches before choosing which to pursue.

Because microdeletions or duplications are not associated with AMA, younger women are more likely to have a fetus with a microdeletion or duplication (1% −1.7%) than with Down syndrome (.13%). In a study of 2779 fetuses with an aCGH performed, 44% of the findings on array were not detectable by cell-free DNA screening (ie, were not trisomies 21, 18, or 13; monosomy X; or a sex chromosome trisomy).[31] This is an important consideration when a pregnant woman is deciding between screening and diagnostic testing. In addition, women older than 35 years and those with a positive biochemical and/or nuchal translucency test still retain a risk of CNVs or rare trisomy results, despite a negative cell-free DNA screen.

Cell-Free DNA Screening and Microdeletions

To address the importance of CNVs and rare cytogenetic abnormalities, laboratories have begun developing the ability to identify smaller cytogenetic changes using cell-free DNA. Currently, some of the available cell-free DNA platforms screen for a limited number (5–7) of previously selected and well-phenotyped microdeletion syndromes. This is the approach used by laboratories in which cell-free DNA screening is done by targeted sequence analysis. (See discussion of Brian L. Shaffer and Mary E. Norton's article, "Cell-Free DNA Screening for Aneuploidy and Microdeletion/Duplication Syndromes," in this issue.) In this case, multiple closely placed probes within the areas of the desired deletions are required. Alternatively, for those using massively parallel shotgun sequencing, deeper sequencing is used to identify alterations in smaller regions of the genome. This approach is limited by the cost and time required for such sequencing. This method has the ability identify CNVs throughout the genome but only diagnose those greater than a prespecified size (usually 5–7 Mb).[32] Because many CNVs are smaller than 5 Mb, specific regions associated with known syndromes may also be targeted to identify CNVs less than 5 Mb in these regions. The detection rates of cell-free DNA screening for CNVs vary dramatically depending on the platform, laboratory, region, and size of the deletion or duplication.

Because, individually, the common microdeletions occur much less often (1/34000 or less) than Down syndrome, the positive predictive value for any is low, leading to a significant number of false-positive results. This becomes even more significant when screening for multiple rare CNVs or performing genomewide CNV screening. One way to address this is to have a very high specificity for any event, which will come at the expense of sensitivity. Despite the false-positive rates required for a clinically appropriate sensitivity, the positive predictive value or likelihood that a positive is a true positive, is still much lower for CNVs than it is for trisomy 21.

Currently, there is insufficient information on the performance of cell-free DNA screening for microdeletions when used for population screening. Accordingly, most societies, including the ACOG, the SMFM, the European Society for Human Genetics, and the American Society for Human Genetics, do not recommend it.[33,34] ACMG on the other hand, recommends informing women of the availability of screening for select microdeletions (but not whole genome) when specific conditions are met by both the provider and the laboratory.[35]

COUNSELING CONSIDERATION

Pretest and posttest counseling about CMA should be performed by a genetic counselor, geneticist, or other provider with expertise in CMA.[11]

Pretest Counseling

Pretest counseling should address the testing options available, the patient's assessment of risk and benefits, and their personal beliefs and attitudes about parenting a child with disabilities.[36] Benefits and limitations should be reviewed before testing, including the potential for identification of consanguinity and nonpaternity.[11] Patients should understand the type and variability of potential results they could be given from CMA, such as early-onset severe conditions, susceptibility to autism and schizophrenia, and later onset less severe disorders, which may be unrelated to the indication for testing. Rather than review the broad list of conditions, the focus should lie on the types of conditions with specific examples. It should be clear that some of these findings may also be found in parents of affected children, some of whom are mildly affected and unaware of any clinical problem. The patient should understand the likelihood of finding a significant CNV based on their referral indication. Specific discussion should occur that addresses the chance of identifying a variant of uncertain significance for which little to no information may be available or a finding with significant variability in which the clinical spectrum of the disorder may not be predictable. Finally, patients should be informed that microarray cannot detect all genetic alterations and that a normal CMA does not rule out the possibility of a genetic condition or birth defect in the pregnancy and the background risk still remains at 2% to 3%.

van der Steen and colleagues[37] evaluated whether pregnant women have sufficient knowledge to make an informed choice about higher versus lower resolution microarray testing on their fetus. They found that women who opted for broader coverage (0.5 Mb) made informed choices significantly more often than women who opted for less coverage (5 Mb). Knowing the potential outcomes, the women preferred to gain information about susceptibility loci in their unborn child. Unlike previous research, which focuses on making sure the woman has sufficient knowledge to make a choice, this study also focuses on attitude consistency and gives the recommendation that the choice a woman makes about the scope of genetic testing on their pregnancy should fit their personal values. They suggest, therefore, that attitude and values should be explored and discussed as a part of pretest counseling, in addition to the goal of increasing the knowledge about the test.

Posttest Counseling

Variants of uncertain significance (VOUS) results are generally reported to patients. The likelihood of such a result varies depending on the coverage of the platform, especially across the backbone. Hillman and colleagues[25] report a VOUS rate of 1.4% when all indications are considered. This is consistent with a Wapner and colleagues[6] study that initially suggested a 1.5% rate of VOUS. However, with time and accumulated data, the implications of many of these have now been better defined. VOUS requires research in advance of the appointment for the medical provider and additional counseling time for the patient. Recent SMFM guidelines suggest that patients with results of uncertain significance should receive counseling from an expert that can review and discuss potentially genotype-phenotype correlations as found on available databases.[11]

Initial studies at the time of introduction of CMA showed that many women chose microarray because the increased information available was an offer too good to pass up. However, in cases in which uncertain or abnormal results were discovered, some felt blindsided and unprepared, and 1 thought the knowledge was toxic.[38] Most informative was the comment that they needed support beyond the time of the initial diagnosis. These comments support the importance of the posttest care.

If a patient has a result of known clinical significance or a VOUS, they should be referred for genetic counseling or for consultation with a geneticist. The session with the patient should review the finding; associated abnormalities and disease course; available published information and case reports; additional testing in the parents or other family members, if appropriate; additional testing in the fetus, such as fetal echocardiogram and ultrasound, as indicated; and the pregnancy options available. Referrals to pediatric genetics or other specialists, and introductions to support groups and other families with a child who has the same condition, can be useful in helping the patient comprehend the diagnosis and make a decision about the pregnancy. Follow-up with the patient on the telephone or in person should occur.

SUMMARY

CMA has the ability to identify microdeletions and duplications too small to be seen on standard karyotype analysis. These CNVs of known clinical significance occur in 1% to 1.7% of pregnancies and are not associated with maternal age. In pregnancies with ultrasound anomalies, clinically significant CNVs are seen in approximately 6%. Accordingly, CMA is the recommended standard of care for all pregnancies undergoing invasive testing after identification of an ultrasound abnormality. Those having invasive testing for other indications, such as maternal age, anxiety, and abnormal serum screening, should routinely be offered microarray as an option. Clinicians ordering CMA should be familiar with the different technologies and laboratory reporting practices. For any patient pursuing CMA, pretest counseling is imperative for them to understand the benefits and limitations, and to make an appropriate decision regarding testing. For patients with abnormal CMA results, including those with VOUS, posttest counseling should be in-depth and be conducted by a genetic counselor or geneticist.

REFERENCES

1. Miller DT, Adam MP, Aradhya S, et al. Consensus statement: chromosomal microarray is a first-tier clinical diagnostic test for individuals with developmental disabilities or congenital anomalies. Am J Hum Genet 2010;86(5):749–64.
2. Fan YS, Jayakar P, Zhu H, et al. Detection of pathogenic gene copy number variations in patients with mental retardation by genomewide oligonucleotide array comparative genomic hybridization. Hum Mutat 2007;28(11):1124–32.
3. American College of Obstetricians and Gynecologists Committee on Genetics. Committee opinion No. 581: the use of chromosomal microarray analysis in prenatal diagnosis. Obstet Gynecol 2013;122(6):1374–7.
4. American College of Obstetricians and Gynecologists. ACOG Practice Bulletin No. 88, December 2007. Invasive prenatal testing for aneuploidy. Obstet Gynecol 2007;110(6):1459–67.
5. American College of Obstetricians and Gynecologists' Committee on Practice Bulletins—Obstetrics, Committee on GeneticsSociety for Maternal–Fetal Medicine. Practice Bulletin No. 162: prenatal diagnostic testing for genetic disorders. Obstet Gynecol 2016;127(5):e108–22.
6. Wapner RJ, Martin CL, Levy B, et al. Chromosomal microarray versus karyotyping for prenatal diagnosis. N Engl J Med 2012;367(23):2175–84.
7. Coppinger J, Alliman S, Lamb AN, et al. Whole-genome microarray analysis in prenatal specimens identifies clinically significant chromosome alterations without increase in results of unclear significance compared to targeted microarray. Prenat Diagn 2009;29(12):1156–66.

8. Richards S, Aziz N, Bale S, et al. Standards and guidelines for the interpretation of sequence variants: a joint consensus recommendation of the American College of Medical Genetics and genomics and the association for molecular pathology. Genet Med 2015;17(5):405–24.

9. Kearney HM, Thorland EC, Brown KK, et al. American College of Medical Genetics standards and guidelines for interpretation and reporting of postnatal constitutional copy number variants. Genet Med 2011;13(7):680–5.

10. South ST, Lee C, Lamb AN, et al. ACMG standards and guidelines for constitutional cytogenomic microarray analysis, including postnatal and prenatal applications: revision 2013. Genet Med 2013;15(11):901–9.

11. Dugoff L, Norton ME, Kuller JA. The use of chromosomal microarray for prenatal diagnosis. Am J Obstet Gynecol 2016;215(4):B2–9.

12. Hook EB. Exclusion of chromosomal mosaicism: tables of 90%, 95% and 99% confidence limits and comments on use. Am J Hum Genet 1977;29(1):94–7.

13. Srebniak MI, Joosten M, Knapen M, et al. Frequency of submicroscopic chromosome aberrations in pregnancies without increased risk for structural chromosome aberrations: a systematic review of literature and meta-analysis. Ultrasound Obstet Gynecol 2017. [Epub ahead of print].

14. Wapner RJ, Zachary J, Clifton R. Change in classification of prenatal microarray analysis copy number variants over time [abstract]. Prenatal Diagnosis 2015; 35(Supplement S1):1–26.

15. Van Opstal D, de Vries F, Govaerts L, et al. Benefits and burdens of using a SNP array in pregnancies at increased risk for the common aneuploidies. Hum Mutat 2015;36(3):319–26.

16. Bornstein E, Berger S, Cheung SW, et al. Universal prenatal chromosomal microarray analysis: additive value and clinical dilemmas in fetuses with a normal karyotype. Am J Perinatol 2017;34(4):340–8.

17. Shaffer LG, Dabell MP, Fisher AJ, et al. Experience with microarray-based comparative genomic hybridization for prenatal diagnosis in over 5000 pregnancies. Prenat Diagn 2012;32(10):976–85.

18. Scott F, Murphy K, Carey L, et al. Prenatal diagnosis using combined quantitative fluorescent polymerase chain reaction and array comparative genomic hybridization analysis as a first-line test: results from over 1000 consecutive cases. Ultrasound Obstet Gynecol 2013;41(5):500–7.

19. Callaway JL, Shaffer LG, Chitty LS, et al. The clinical utility of microarray technologies applied to prenatal cytogenetics in the presence of a normal conventional karyotype: a review of the literature. Prenat Diagn 2013;33(12):1119–23.

20. Le Vaillant C, Beneteau C, Chan-Leconte N, et al. [Beckwith-Wiedemann syndrome: What do you search in prenatal diagnosis? about 14 cases]. Gynecol Obstet Fertil 2015;43(11):705–11.

21. Wax JR, Burroughs R, Wright MS. Prenatal sonographic features of Russell-Silver syndrome. J Ultrasound Med 1996;15(3):253–5.

22. Committee opinion No.682: microarrays and next-generation sequencing technology: the use of advanced genetic diagnostic tools in obstetrics and gynecology. Obstet Gynecol 2016;128(6):e262–8.

23. Reddy UM, Page GP, Saade GR, et al. Karyotype versus microarray testing for genetic abnormalities after stillbirth. N Engl J Med 2012;367(23):2185–93.

24. Srebniak MI, Diderich KE, Joosten M, et al. Prenatal SNP array testing in 1000 fetuses with ultrasound anomalies: causative, unexpected and susceptibility CNVs. Eur J Hum Genet 2016;24(5):645–51.

25. Hillman SC, McMullan DJ, Hall G, et al. Use of prenatal chromosomal microarray: prospective cohort study and systematic review and meta-analysis. Ultrasound Obstet Gynecol 2013;41(6):610–20.
26. Shaffer LG, Coppinger J, Alliman S, et al. Comparison of microarray-based detection rates for cytogenetic abnormalities in prenatal and neonatal specimens. Prenat Diagn 2008;28(9):789–95.
27. Kleeman L, Bianchi DW, Shaffer LG, et al. Use of array comparative genomic hybridization for prenatal diagnosis of fetuses with sonographic anomalies and normal metaphase karyotype. Prenat Diagn 2009;29(13):1213–7.
28. Faas BH, van der Burgt I, Kooper AJ, et al. Identification of clinically significant, submicroscopic chromosome alterations and UPD in fetuses with ultrasound anomalies using genome-wide 250k SNP array analysis. J Med Genet 2010; 47(9):586–94.
29. Shaffer LG, Rosenfeld JA, Dabell MP, et al. Detection rates of clinically significant genomic alterations by microarray analysis for specific anomalies detected by ultrasound. Prenat Diagn 2012;32(10):986–95.
30. Donnelly JC, Platt LD, Rebarber A, et al. Association of copy number variants with specific ultrasonographically detected fetal anomalies. Obstet Gynecol 2014; 124(1):83–90.
31. Sotiriadis A, Papoulidis I, Siomou E, et al. Non-invasive prenatal screening versus prenatal diagnosis by array comparative genomic hybridization: a comparative retrospective study. Prenat Diagn 2017;37(6):583–92.
32. Lefkowitz RB, Tynan JA, Liu T, et al. Clinical validation of a noninvasive prenatal test for genomewide detection of fetal copy number variants. Am J Obstet Gynecol 2016;215(2):227.e1–16.
33. Dondorp W, de Wert G, Bombard Y, et al. Non-invasive prenatal testing for aneuploidy and beyond: challenges of responsible innovation in prenatal screening. Summary and recommendations. Eur J Hum Genet 2015. [Epub ahead of print].
34. Committee opinion summary No. 640: cell-free DNA screening for fetal aneuploidy. Obstet Gynecol 2015;126(3):691–2.
35. Gregg AR, Skotko BG, Benkendorf JL, et al. Noninvasive prenatal screening for fetal aneuploidy, 2016 update: a position statement of the American College of Medical Genetics and Genomics. Genet Med 2016;18(10):1056–65.
36. Fonda Allen J, Stoll K, Bernhardt BA. Pre- and post-test genetic counseling for chromosomal and Mendelian disorders. Semin Perinatol 2016;40(1):44–55.
37. van der Steen SL, Bunnik EM, Polak MG, et al. Choosing between higher and lower resolution microarrays: do pregnant women have sufficient knowledge to make informed choices consistent with their attitude? J Genet Couns 2017. [Epub ahead of print].
38. Bernhardt BA, Soucier D, Hanson K, et al. Women's experiences receiving abnormal prenatal chromosomal microarray testing results. Genet Med 2013; 15(2):139–45.

Whole Exome Sequencing
Applications in Prenatal Genetics

Angie C. Jelin, MD[a], Neeta Vora, MD[b],*

KEYWORDS

- Fetal • Exome • Sequencing • Prenatal ultrasonography • Abnormalities

KEY POINTS

- Prenatal whole exome sequencing is emerging as a valuable tool for fetal diagnosis in the setting of sonographic abnormalities.
- Diagnostic rates are variable across studies, with improved rates when trio (proband, mother father) whole exome sequencing is performed.
- Prenatal genetic counseling is crucial for appropriate parental consent for whole exome sequencing.
- There are many ethical considerations, including risks of discrimination, that must be considered when whole exome sequencing is performed.

BACKGROUND

Ultrasonography-detected fetal sonographic abnormalities are identified in 2% to 3% of pregnancies.[1] Genetic diagnosis with amniocentesis or chorionic villus sampling with chromosomal microarray (CMA) and karyotype are routinely offered in these cases. Of cases that undergo diagnostic testing, a karyotype abnormality is found in 8% to 10% of cases, whereas a microdeletion/duplication is identified in another 6%, leaving most families without a specific genetic diagnosis.[2] These families must therefore be counseled based on ultrasonography findings alone. Management decisions thus need to be made from limited information and counseling is challenging because of the broad differential diagnosis and large range of prognoses and expectations. Whole exome sequencing (WES), rather than targeted disease-specific gene panels, is now being studied and used to improve prenatal diagnosis in cases in which structural abnormalities are identified sonographically. Initial studies show that prenatal WES can elucidate the responsible pathogenic variants in an additional 20%[3] to

Disclosures: None.
[a] Division of Maternal-Fetal Medicine, Department of Gynecology and Obstetrics, Johns Hopkins School of Medicine, 500 North Wolfe Street, Phipps 222, Baltimore, MD 21218, USA;
[b] Division of Maternal-Fetal Medicine, Department of Obstetrics and Gynecology, University of North Carolina at Chapel Hill, 3010 Old Clinic Building/Cb# 7516, Chapel Hill, NC 27599, USA
* Corresponding author.
E-mail address: neeta_vora@med.unc.edu

Obstet Gynecol Clin N Am 45 (2018) 69–81
https://doi.org/10.1016/j.ogc.2017.10.003
0889-8545/18/© 2017 Elsevier Inc. All rights reserved.

80%[4] of cases when standard genetic testing (karyotype and CMA) is normal. The diagnostic yield of prenatal WES is known to be highly dependent on the indication for WES.

WES, unlike whole genome sequencing (WGS), is currently clinically available and focuses on the exons or protein coding regions of the genome only (**Fig. 1**). Exons account for 1.5%[5] of the DNA in the genome, comprising approximately 22,000 genes. Most identified genes implicated in mendelian disease involve the exons.[6] Thus, WES is more cost-effective than WGS. In addition, WES is preferred because the ability to interpret intronic regions of the genome is currently extremely limited. Prenatal WES has the ability to increase diagnostic rates in cases in which fetal anomalies are present and enhance the understanding of pathogenic variants that are developmentally lethal.[7] WES also has the potential to expand known disease phenotypes to the prenatal period. Multiple challenges of prenatal WES include (1) interpreting the vast amount of data in a timely manner; (2) identifying pathogenic variants in diseases with reduced penetrance and variable expressivity; and (3) providing adequate pretest and posttest counseling, particularly with regard to the stress/uncertainly associated with discovering variants of unknown significance (VUS).[8]

Prenatal WES has the potential to increase the ability to provide a more precise diagnosis, which will then improve the ability to counsel families. It is also often the first step in improving the path toward informed diagnosis and treatment, which is especially important in the era of advancing in utero fetal therapy. This article discusses the current literature regarding prenatal WES, clinical indications for WES, challenges with interpretation/counseling (VUS), research priorities, ethical issues, and potential future advances.

PRENATAL

As of July 2017, the prenatal data for exome sequencing currently includes 16 case series with 5 or more fetuses (7 articles and 9 conference abstracts) and several

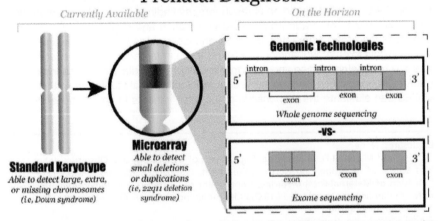

Fig. 1. New genomic technologies such as whole genome and whole exome sequencing have the ability to interrogate the fetal genome more comprehensively than currently available tests. (*From* Hardisty EE, Vora NL. Advances in genetic prenatal diagnosis and screening. Curr Opin Pediatr 2014;26(6):635; with permission.)

additional case reports.[9] The overall diagnostic rate ranges from 6.2%[10] to 57.1% (**Table 1**)[11] in published articles and up to 80% when abstracts are included.[4,9] The diagnostic rate depends on the indication for WES and varies based on multiple factors, including single versus multiple organ system affected, specific organ system affected, and proband versus trio sequencing. The lowest reported rate of 6.2% was obtained by performing WES on all fetuses with any anomaly visualized on ultrasonography, whereas the highest rates were in small studies with carefully chosen cases.[11–13] WES was successful in determining the diagnosis in 3.6% to 6.2% of isolated anomalies and 14.3% to 16% of fetuses with ultrasonography findings affecting multiple organ systems.[10] Certain organ systems seem to have a higher yield of reported pathogenic variants. For example, in a cohort of 84 deceased fetuses, a pathogenic variant was identified by WES more frequently in fetuses with isolated neurologic abnormalities compared with those with isolated cardiovascular findings (37% vs 31%).[14] The yield is also increased when WES is performed on a trio (maternal, paternal, proband).[15] The use of trios allows the prioritization of review of variants that have an increased likelihood of being pathogenic using a standard analytical framework that takes into account potential de novo variants (present in fetus but absent from the parents) or recessively inherited variants (homozygous or compound heterozygous in the fetus and heterozygous in parents).

Table 1
Fetal exome sequencing published case series

First Author	Number of Cases	Cohort Description	Proband vs Trio	Pathogenic Variant	Likely Pathogenic Variant
Yang et al,[12] 2014	11	Terminated anomalous fetuses	Trio	6 out of 11 (54%)	—
Carss et al,[15] 2014	30	Prenatal sonographic anomalies	Trio	3 out of 30 (10%)	5 out of 30 (16.7%)
Drury et al,[3] 2015	24	Prenatal sonographic anomalies including NT ≥3.5 mm	14 Proband 10 Trio	5 out of 24 (20.8%)	1 out of 24 (4.2%)
Alamillo et al,[11] 2015	7	Multiple sonographic anomalies termination or demise	Trio	3 out of 7 (42.9%)	1 out of 7 (14.3%)
Pangalos et al,[13] 2016	14	Prenatal sonographic anomalies	Proband only	6 out of 14 (42.9%)	—
Yates et al,[14] 2017	84	Demise or termination	33 Proband/duo 51 Trio/quad	17 out of 84 (20%)	38 out of 84 (45%)
Vora et al,[26] 2017	15	Multiple sonographic anomalies	Trio	7 out of 15 (46.7%)	1 out of 15 (6.7%)

Abbreviation: NT, nuchal translucency.

The outcomes of a prenatal diagnosis can be extreme, and require significant counseling with regard to reproductive decision making.[16] When the pregnancy is continued, the diagnosis can assist with palliative care decisions, including comfort care, or a diagnosis can inform the pediatricians about management or possible treatments that may be offered postnatally. A diagnosis with WES may also reduce hospital costs by decreasing the number of tests performed postnatally, thereby avoiding the so-called diagnostic odyssey and potentially decreasing the length of the hospital stay.[17,18] When performed clinically in the prenatal or neonatal period, a positive result can have implications for other family members and/or for future pregnancies. In a subsequent pregnancy, preimplantation genetic diagnosis could be performed or the patient could have diagnostic testing by chorionic villus sampling or amniocentesis. Understanding the genetic cause can also provide closure for the families and help with the grieving process in cases of fetal or neonatal loss.[19]

Many mendelian disorders do not have a known prenatal phenotype and the molecular diagnosis may not be suspected because the phenotype may be atypical from what is described postnatally. Use of prenatal WES has the ability to expand phenotypes to the prenatal period and increase the understanding of genes that may be critical to human development.

Patient preferences and understanding of prenatal genetic diagnosis are extremely variable and likely affect the psychosocial impact of the relayed results. Preference to undergo testing and the desire to make decisions based on the results vary by ethnicity,[20–22] socioeconomic status, cultural and religious beliefs, acceptability of termination of pregnancy, and experiences with disability.[23–25] Vora and colleagues[26] found in a pilot study on prenatal WES that women with lower family incomes scored significantly lower on the genetics literacy assessment compared with women with higher family incomes. They also found that women with lower family incomes (<$50,000 vs >$89,999) had increased expectations that WES would provide a reason for the fetal abnormalities (Likert scale, 5.2 out of 10) despite appropriate pretest counseling by a genetic counselor about an approximate 30% diagnostic yield. Further research on this critical topic of patient expectations and understanding is needed to ensure that patients' needs are being met as new technologies inevitably become implemented into clinical practice.

Therapy

Fetal intervention to treat genetic disease has been in use for more than 50 decades. One of the earliest uses of in utero therapy is intrauterine transfusions for fetal rhesus isoimmunization.[27] In the era of advanced fetal therapy, including in utero myelomeningocele repair, fetal cardiac intervention,[28] fetal endotracheal occlusion for congenital diaphragmatic hernia (CDH), and potentially in utero amnioinfusion for bilateral renal agenesis,[29] additional knowledge of the underlying genetic cause of the defect is invaluable.[30] For example, an in utero CDH repair may be less effective in fetuses with syndromic CDH than isolated CDH. It has been proposed[31] that in utero fetal intracerebral shunts could effectively treat severe fetal ventriculomegaly.[32,33] In boys, isolated severe fetal ventriculomegaly is secondary to an *L1CAM* mutation in 2% to 15% of cases.[34] These infants have more severe neurodevelopmental outcomes than other infants with apparently isolated severe ventriculomegaly.[35] It may therefore be reasonable to exclude fetuses with L1CAM mutations or perform subgroup analyses on these infants when trials evaluating the utility of fetal intervention for this condition are performed. This example can be extrapolated to other inherited causes of fetal anomalies. It has yet to be determined whether or not certain underlying genetic conditions may benefit more or less from fetal intervention. Prenatal WES should be studied in cases in which fetal intervention is possible or planned so that further information about best surgical candidates can be obtained.

Until recently, there were few recognizable fetal phenotypes for which evaluation of single-gene mutations were routinely performed. Prenatal molecular diagnosis of specific skeletal dysplasias can often be made with targeted panel testing.[36] However, because of the broad phenotypic spectrum of skeletal and other conditions and the limited information obtained with prenatal ultrasonography, WES may be more efficient and cost-effective. New fetal therapies are currently emerging and are showing improved outcomes in specific skeletal dysplasias.[37] Particularly promising is teriparatide for treatment of osteogenesis imperfecta (OI).[38] The only current in utero therapy for OI is in utero mesenchymal stem cell transplant via the fetal umbilical vein.[39] A transient decrease in fractures has been shown in case series.[40] The BOOSTB4 (Boost Brittle Bones Before Birth) study is a feasibility study that is underway to study the use of stem cell transplant in 15 cases of OI with in utero diagnosis.[41] As additional postnatal therapies for genetic syndromes evolve, their application to fetal life will need to be explored. Thus, application of prenatal WES to such cases may help identify which pregnancies would benefit most from in utero therapies.

CLINICAL INDICATIONS

WES is recommended in pediatric and adult medicine for clinical indications such as multiple birth defects or neurodevelopmental delay when other tests have been uninformative. Postnatal data show an overall diagnostic yield of 25% to 30%, depending on the affected organ system.[12,42] The American College of Medical Genetics and Genomics (ACMG) recommends WES when a genetic disorder is suggested by phenotype and family history and either targeted genetic testing is not available or available testing performed is not diagnostic.[43] It is both current practice and cost-effective to perform a microarray before WES. Experts also suggest performing targeted testing before WES when a specific syndrome is suspected. If the presenting disorder is highly genetically heterogeneous, WES is potentially more cost-effective than sequencing individual genes.[44]

ACMG and the Society of Maternal-Fetal Medicine (SMFM) recommend that all patients considering WES receive counseling from a provider with genetics expertise. However, given that WES is in its infancy and studies are ongoing to determine its clinical utility, ACMG and SMFM do not recommend WES for routine use for prenatal diagnosis.[45]

In select cases in which other approaches to diagnosis have been uninformative, it may be appropriate to offer WES. Examples of such cases include recurrent or multiple congenital anomalies, heterotaxy, and undiagnosed skeletal dysplasias. Prenatal WES also has a role in cases in which a fetus has structural abnormalities with reported consanguinity or homozygosity indicating relatedness on microarray.

American College of Medical Genetics and Genomics Reportable Variants

The current ACMG reporting recommendations include not only reporting the clinically relevant findings that could be contributing to the primary phenotype for which the testing was requested but also offering reports of secondary findings for medical conditions that are potentially medically actionable. Secondary findings include pathogenic variants in genes responsible for conditions that are unrelated to the indication for which testing was initially performed. The initial ACMG recommendation included mandatory reporting of specified variants in 56 genes.[46] ACMG recently modified the recommendations to optional reporting, removing 4 genes and adding an additional gene, resulting in reporting recommendations for 59 genes.[47] ACMG recommends reporting only known pathogenic or disease-causing variants within the genes and not benign variants. Literature suggests that WES identifies a secondary finding in 1% of cases.[48] Most reportable incidental variants occur in genes responsible for a predisposition to cancer or a cardiac event. The clinical treatment modalities for these variants have variable efficacy and are currently far from curative.

Before these ACMGs guidelines, societies did not recommend testing children for adult-onset diseases until they reached sufficient maturity to provide informed consent.[49] The incidental variant guidelines created a paradigm shift, recommending parents opt out of receiving information about secondary findings identified on WES of their child or fetus.

INTERPRETATION/COUNSELING

Pretest and posttest counseling are recommended for all prenatal genetic screening and diagnostic testing. Ideally, both the mother and father are present for the counseling session. A trained professional with genetics expertise should obtain complete clinical information along with a 3-generation pedigree. Specifically, when taking a pedigree in a prenatal genetics clinic, the fetus and any siblings, miscarriages, or fetal losses should be included in 1 of these 3 generations. Testing should be ordered only by specialists who are comfortable with the interpretation and explanation of results. Information should include options for reproductive decision making, pregnancy, and perinatal management.[50]

There are risks, benefits, and limitations to every form of prenatal screening or diagnosis. There are 5 specific items that should be mentioned during pretest counseling for prenatal WES. The results of the testing could provide the following information:

1. A primary finding could be identified or suggested to explain the fetal phenotype. This primary finding includes variants in genes that could explain the medical conditions for which the testing is being performed.
2. A negative result for which a diagnosis is not available for the phenotype in question.
3. A variant of unknown significance (VOUS), which may or may not be related to the condition for which the testing is obtained.
4. A secondary or incidental finding could be identified, which refers to a pathogenic variant in a gene that causes a genetic condition, unrelated to the indication for testing.
5. Genetic relationships could be identified, including the identification of false paternity or consanguinity.

Patients undergoing prenatal WES need appropriate informed consent to make decisions about opting in or out of receiving information on VOUS and secondary/incidental findings. In addition to the 5 statements listed earlier, patients should also be informed that the knowledge of variants is continuously evolving so an unreported variant, or a variant that is coded as unknown in significance at the time WES is initially performed, may be found to be pathogenic in the future. Primary or secondary gene mutations identified in the fetus could also have impacts on the patient's health, other family members' health, and future pregnancies.

VOUS are particularly problematic in the prenatal setting.[51] Providers who offer and counsel about prenatal microarray have experience with counseling patients regarding uncertain results. Laboratories performing WES often provide limited reports to decrease the number of VOUS reported to the clinician. Herein lies the ethical balance of reporting and counseling. Current databases such as ClinVar,[52] Human Genetics Mutation Database,[53] and Exome Aggregation Consortium[54] include limited fetal phenotypic data, making fetal phenotypes especially challenging to interpret.

The interpretation of WES is simple when a previously reported pathogenic mutation with a well-documented phenotype is identified. The most critical data to arrive at the correct diagnosis involve phenotypic data from ultrasonography, fetal MRI (if performed), and fetal autopsy. However, detailed phenotypic information is not often available prenatally. Thus, a definitive diagnosis cannot be made in many cases. Instead, multiple variants are identified and must be filtered using pipelines specific to trios along with whatever phenotypic data are available to determine possible pathogenicity. Laboratories and clinics should have clear guidelines and policies related to reporting of findings and all reported variants should be confirmed with Sanger sequencing because false-positive results can occur with WES given that sequencing of many fragments occurs simultaneously. Databases with phenotypic and molecular data (ClinGen/ClinVar) currently do not have a prenatal component. However, given that WES is starting to be used prenatally in select cases, it is critical that a shared prenatal database become available to further understand genotype/phenotype correlations prenatally and to enable clinicians and researchers to determine whether the variants found in their patients were seen in other patients with the same phenotype.

LIMITATIONS

Although WES is performed to evaluate single nucleotide variants in expressed areas of the genome, it has many limitations. Some of the limitations can be overcome by increasing the depth of sequencing, whereas others are inherent defects of the current technology. WES does not detect differences in copy number variation, for which microarray technology is required. It is not designed to detect aneuploidy (ie, trisomy 21), polyploidy (ie, triploidy, tetraploidy), nor does it detect translocations, trinucleotide repeats (repeat expansions, tandem repeat size), or low-level mosaicism. There are several regions in the genome with poor depth/coverage, particularly guanine-cytosine (GC)–rich areas,[55] that are not adequately sequenced with WES. Sanger sequencing is recommended to verify all reported results.

In addition to the overall challenges of WES, the long turnaround time is especially problematic in the prenatal setting. Limited anatomy can be visualized on sonogram before the anatomic survey performed at 18 to 22 weeks' gestation. In addition, primary testing with microarray or panel testing is generally performed before sending WES. When performed rapidly, results can be obtained within 2 to 3 weeks. It is anticipated that the turnaround will become faster and more cost-effective over time.[56]

RESEARCH IMPLICATIONS

Several National Institutes of Health (NIH)–funded centers are currently performing WES for the purpose of identification of novel genes. Initiation of WES was quickly followed by an increase in the discovery of the known function of genes.[57] Most novel genes are identified postnatally; however, genes responsible for lethal fetal conditions or recurrent miscarriages rely on prenatal WES and WGS to provide insight into the function of genes that may be critical to human development.

It is critical that researchers performing prenatal WES be committed to sharing data. A common database for prenatal phenotypes with molecular findings by WES is essential to optimizing clinical care. Data sharing is recommended for clinical laboratories as well as researchers. The NIH requires grant submitters to supply information on their current plans, including patient consent, to participate in genome-wide data sharing. Centers are often willing to perform WES on patients with specific fetal defects; for example, the DHREAMS (Diaphragmatic Hernia Research & Exploration; Advancing Molecular Science) study[58] based at Columbia University Medical Center will perform WES on patients with CDH seen at other centers.

ETHICS

Multiple ethical issues associated with prenatal WES have been brought to attention.[59] Of primary concern to patients are adequate interpretation and disclosure of appropriate variants. Interpretation and disclosure are particularly important in the prenatal period, when the decision to continue a pregnancy could be determined by the reported variant. In addition, patient counseling requires appropriate consent and disclosure of secondary and incidental variants, recontact for reclassification of variants, discussion of informing affected family members, loss of privacy associated with data sharing, as well as potential discrimination if a genetic diagnosis is made.

Genetic professionals have an ethical obligation to follow appropriate protocols for patient consent[60] and interpretation of variants. It is particularly important to discuss the options of opting in or out of receiving information on secondary/incidental findings and VOUS.[61] In the case of trio analysis, it is essential to consent the mother separately from the father to discuss that nonpaternity may be disclosed from prenatal WES. She would then have an option to opt out of testing. Patients should consider all testing options available, including panel testing when appropriate. In the future, and potentially even now, WES could be more cost-effective than panel testing; however, WES can result in a significant amount of unintended information.

An ethical dilemma inherent in genetic testing is ensuring that genetic information remains confidential.[62] This confidentiality is confounded by the importance of data sharing in the understanding and classification of variants. Efforts have been made to limit potential discrimination secondary to results. The Genetic Information Nondiscrimination Act of 2008 prevents the use of genetic information for health insurance. It does not, however, apply to life, disability, long-term-care, or certain federal employee health care programs.

Challenges of interpretation and reporting remain barriers to widespread use of prenatal WES. Molecular geneticists and molecular variant analysts are responsible for maximizing reporting of positives while minimizing the reporting of potentially benign variants. Regardless of this balance, until comprehensive WES data are deposited in publicly available databases, false-negatives and false-positives will be reported.

COSTS

Most of the cost of performing WES is represents the costs of variant analysis. Well-trained molecular variant analysts or molecular geneticists are essential to providing accurate results. Most clinical and research laboratories have committees made of multidisciplinary teams to review the findings from prenatal WES. These teams may include molecular geneticists, cytogeneticists, clinical geneticists, genetic counselors, bioethicists, and bioinformaticians. In addition to accurately interpreting and reporting primary findings that explain the fetal phenotype, it is essential to interpret and report secondary findings, presuming that consent was obtained from the patients to receive such findings. A system for reanalysis and reevaluation of variants over time is also necessary because genes whose functions were previously unknown are being discovered and categorized at a rapid rate. Sanger sequencing is also recommended for confirmation of variants for the patients and for the family members who receive results about medically actionable findings that were unrelated to the fetal phenotype, such as any of the ACMG-specified variants in 59 genes.[45] Costs will presumably decrease as technology advances and interpretation algorithms improve.

Although a diagnosis is thought to be cost-effective, it often does incur medical costs, including additional recommended medical screening, evaluation, and or therapy related to the diagnosis for either the patient and/or family members. There is also an emotional cost associated with having a test performed whether the result is positive, negative, or VOUS.[63]

FUTURE ADVANCES

WES and WGS are rapidly evolving with advances in research and technology. The ability to perform WGS has quickly followed WES and is currently being studied on a research basis. The limitations of interpretation of WES seem minor compared with interpretation challenges of WGS data.[64] There will likely be a pivotal point in the future at which cost and knowledge will make WGS more cost-effective and widely performed.

In addition, advances in prenatal screening, including cell-free DNA (cfDNA), have reduced the use of chorionic villus sampling and amniocentesis. cfDNA technology allows the detection of cell-free placental DNA in maternal blood and is a clinically recommended screening method for women who are at high risk for having a pregnancy affected with a common aneuploidy.[65] Capabilities of performing WES on cfDNA currently exist.[66,67] As technology improves and cost decreases, it is likely that WES using cfDNA will be clinically available. Some of the limitations of this technology will persist, including that the cells in the maternal system are derived from trophoblasts and are not a pure representation of fetal DNA. When screening tests using cfDNA show an increased risk for a specific diagnosis, a diagnostic test will continue to be necessary to rule out placental mosaicism or other causes of a false-positive screen.

Single-cell technology has been proposed as a more accurate technology than the current cell-free platforms.[68,69] Rather than relying on maternal/fetal ratios, single-cell technology allows a single fetal cell to be specifically evaluated. If used, several cells need to be evaluated to evaluate for sequencing errors or mosaicism. This technology potentially has more promise for cell-free WES than the current noninvasive cell-free technologies secondary to the lack of maternal contamination.

In summary, further research is needed to determine best practices for clinical implementation of WES specifically related to interpretation, turnaround time, and optimal ways to counsel patients given that it is only a matter of time before WES becomes available using noninvasive technologies.

REFERENCES

1. Centers for Disease Control and Prevention (CDC). Update on overall prevalence of major birth defects–Atlanta, Georgia, 1978-2005. MMWR Morb Mortal Wkly Rep 2008;57:1–5.
2. Wapner RJ, Martin CL, Levy B, et al. Chromosomal microarray versus karyotyping for prenatal diagnosis. N Engl J Med 2012;367:2175–84.
3. Drury S, Williams H, Trump N, et al. Exome sequencing for prenatal diagnosis of fetuses with sonographic abnormalities. Prenat Diagn 2015;35:1010–7.
4. Yadava SM, Ashkinadze E. 125: whole exome sequencing (WES) in prenatal diagnosis for carefully selected cases. Am J Obstet Gynecol 2017;216:S87–8.
5. Ng SB, Turner EH, Robertson PD, et al. Targeted capture and massively parallel sequencing of 12 human exomes. Nature 2009;461(7261):272–6.

6. Majewski J, Schwartzentruber J, Lalonde E, et al. What can exome sequencing do for you? J Med Genet 2011;48:580–9.
7. Medeira A, Norman A, Haslam J, et al. Examination of fetuses after induced abortion for fetal abnormality—a follow-up study. Prenat Diagn 1994;14:381–5.
8. Cohen JC, Kiss RS, Pertsemlidis A, et al. Multiple rare alleles contribute to low plasma levels of HDL cholesterol. Science 2004;305(5685):869–72.
9. Best S, Wou K, Vora N, et al. Promises, pitfalls and practicalities of prenatal whole exome sequencing. Prenat Diagn 2017. [Epub ahead of print].
10. Wapner R, Petrovski S, Brennan K, et al. Whole exome sequencing in the evaluation of fetal structural anomalies: a prospective study of sequential patients. Am J Obstet Gynecol 2017;216:S5–6.
11. Alamillo CL, Powis Z, Farwell K, et al. Exome sequencing positively identified relevant alterations in more than half of cases with an indication of prenatal ultrasound anomalies. Prenat Diagn 2015;35:1073–8.
12. Yang Y, Muzny DM, Xia F, et al. Molecular findings among patients referred for clinical whole-exome sequencing. JAMA 2014;312:1807–9.
13. Pangalos C, Hagnefelt B, Lilakos K, et al. First applications of a targeted exome sequencing approach in fetuses with ultrasound abnormalities reveals an important fraction of cases with associated gene defects. PeerJ 2016;4:e1955.
14. Yates CL, Monaghan KG, Copenheaver D, et al. Whole-exome sequencing on deceased fetuses with ultrasound anomalies: expanding our knowledge of genetic disease during fetal development. Genet Med 2017. https://doi.org/10.1038/gim.2017.31.
15. Carss KJ, Hillman SC, Parthiban V, et al. Exome sequencing improves genetic diagnosis of structural fetal abnormalities revealed by ultrasound. Hum Mol Genet 2014;23(12):3269–77.
16. Bernhardt BA, Soucier D, Hanson K, et al. Women's experiences receiving abnormal prenatal chromosomal microarray testing results. Genet Med 2013;15(2):139–45.
17. Valencia CA, Husami A, Holle J, et al. Clinical impact and cost-effectiveness of whole exome sequencing as a diagnostic tool: a pediatric center's experience. Front Pediatr 2015;3:67.
18. Willing LK, Petrikin JE, Smith LD, et al. Whole-genome sequencing for identification of Mendelian disorders in critically ill infants: a retrospective analysis of diagnostic and clinical findings. Lancet Respir Med 2015;3:377–87.
19. Maguire M, Light A, Kuppermann M, et al. Grief after second-trimester termination for fetal anomaly: a qualitative study. Contraception 2015;91(3):234–9.
20. Tschudin S, Huang D, Mor-Gültekin H, et al. Prenatal counseling–implications of the cultural background of pregnant women on information processing, emotional response and acceptance. Ultraschall Med 2011;32(Suppl 2):E100–7.
21. Muhsen K, Na'amnah W, Lesser Y, et al. Determinates of underutilization of amniocentesis among Israeli Arab women. Prenat Diagn 2010;30(2):138–43.
22. Kuppermann M, Learman LA, Gates E, et al. Beyond race or ethnicity and socioeconomic status: predictors of prenatal testing for Down syndrome. Obstet Gynecol 2006;107:1087–97.
23. Case AP, Ramadhani TA, Canfield MA, et al. Awareness and attitudes regarding prenatal testing among Texas women of childbearing age. J Genet Couns 2007;16(5):655–61.
24. Kuppermann M, Gates E, Washington AE. Racial-ethnic differences in prenatal diagnostic test use and outcomes: preferences, socioeconomics, or patient knowledge? Obstet Gynecol 1996;87(5 Pt 1):675–82.

25. Kuppermann M, Nakagawa S, Cohen SR, et al. Attitudes toward prenatal testing and pregnancy termination among a diverse population of parents of children with intellectual disabilities. Prenat Diagn 2011;31(13):1251–8.
26. Vora NL, Powell B, Brandt A, et al. Prenatal exome sequencing in anomalous fetuses: new opportunities and challenges. Genet Med 2017. https://doi.org/10.1038/gim.2017.33.
27. Pattison NS, Roberts AB, Mantell N. Intrauterine fetal transfusion, 1963-90. Ultrasound Obstet Gynecol 1992;2(5):329–32.
28. Moon-Grady AJ, Morris SA, Belfort M, et al. International fetal cardiac intervention registry: a worldwide collaborative description and preliminary outcomes. J Am Coll Cardiol 2015;66(4):388–99.
29. Goebel J. New nephrological frontiers: opportunities and challenges created by fetal care centers. Adv Pediatr 2017;64(1):73–86.
30. McGivern MR, Best KE, Rankin J, et al. Epidemiology of congenital diaphragmatic hernia in Europe: a register-based study. Arch Dis Child Fetal Neonatal Ed 2015;100:F137–44.
31. Chen Y, Emery SP, Maxey AP, et al. A novel low-profile ventriculoamniotic shunt for foetal aqueductal stenosis. J Med Eng Technol 2016;40(4):186–98.
32. Cavalheiro S, da Costa MDS, Mendonça JN, et al. Antenatal management of fetal neurosurgical diseases. Childs Nerv Syst 2017;33(7):1125–41.
33. Cavalheiro S, Moron AF, Zymberg ST, et al. Fetal hydrocephalus—prenatal treatment. Childs Nerv Syst 2003;19:561–73.
34. Kenwrick S, Jouet M, Donnai D. X linked hydrocephalus and MASA syndrome. J Med Genet 1996;33(1):59–65.
35. Stumpel C, Vos YJ. In: Pagon RA, Adam MP, Ardinger HH, et al, editors. L1 Syndrome.GeneReviews®. Seattle (WA): University of Washington; 1993–2017.
36. Chitty LS, Mason S, Barrett AN, et al. Non-invasive prenatal diagnosis of achondroplasia and thanatophoric dysplasia: next generation sequencing allows for a safer, more accurate, and comprehensive approach. Prenat Diagn 2015;35:656–62.
37. Jelin AC, O'Hare E, Blakemore K, et al. Skeletal dysplasias: growing therapy for growing bones. Front Pharmacol 2017;8:79.
38. Orwoll ES, Shapiro J, Veith S, et al. Evaluation of teriparatide treatment in adults with osteogenesis imperfecta. J Clin Invest 2014;124:491–8.
39. Le Blanc K, Götherström C, Ringdén O, et al. Fetal mesenchymal stem-cell engraftment in bone after in utero transplantation in a patient with severe osteogenesis imperfecta. Transplantation 2005;79(11):1607–14.
40. Chan JK, Götherström C. Prenatal transplantation of mesenchymal stem cells to treat osteogenesis imperfecta. Front Pharmacol 2014;5:223.
41. Chitty LS, David AL, Gottschalk I, et al. EP21.04: BOOSTB4: a clinical study to determine safety and efficacy of pre- and/or postnatal stem cell transplantation for treatment of osteogenesis imperfecta. Ultrasound Obstet Gynecol 2016;48(Suppl. 1):356.
42. Deciphering Developmental Disorders Study. Large-scale discovery of novel genetic causes of developmental disorders. Nature 2015;519:223–8.
43. ACMG Board of Directors. Points to consider in the clinical application of genomic sequencing. Genet Med 2012;14(8):759–61.
44. Stark Z, Schofield D, Alam K, et al. Prospective comparison of the cost-effectiveness of clinical whole-exome sequencing with that of usual care overwhelmingly supports early use and reimbursement. Genet Med 2017. https://doi.org/10.1038/gim.2016.221.

45. Committee on Genetics and the Society for Maternal-Fetal Medicine. Committee opinion no.682: microarrays and next-generation sequencing technology: the use of advanced genetic diagnostic tools in obstetrics and gynecology. Obstet Gynecol 2016;128(6):e262–8.
46. Green RC, Berg JS, Grody WW, et al, American College of Medical Genetics and Genomics. ACMG recommendations for reporting of incidental findings in clinical exome and genome sequencing. Genet Med 2013;15(7):565–74.
47. Kalia SS, Adelman K, Bale SJ, et al. Recommendations for reporting of secondary findings in clinical exome and genome sequencing, 2016 update (ACMG SF v2.0): a policy statement of the American College of Medical Genetics and Genomics. Genet Med 2017;19:249–55.
48. Johnston JJ, Rubinstein WS, Facio FM, et al. Secondary variants in individuals undergoing exome sequencing: screening of 572 individuals identifies high-penetrance mutations in cancer-susceptibility genes. Am J Hum Genet 2012;91(1):97–108.
49. Borry P, Evers-Kiebooms G, Cornel MC, et al. Genetic testing in asymptomatic minors. Background considerations towards ESHG recommendations. Eur J Hum Genet 2009;17:711–9.
50. Skirton H, Goldsmith L, Jackson L, et al. Offering prenatal diagnostic tests: European guidelines for clinical practice. Eur J Hum Genet 2014;22:580–6.
51. Westerfield L, Darilek S, van den Veyver IB. Counseling challenges with variants of uncertain significance and incidental findings in prenatal genetic screening and diagnosis. J Clin Med 2014;3:1018–32.
52. Landrum MJ, Lee JM, Benson M, et al. ClinVar: public archive of interpretations of clinically relevant variants. Nucleic Acids Res 2016;44(D1):D862–8.
53. Stenson PD, Mort M, Ball EV, et al. The Human Gene Mutation Database: towards a comprehensive repository of inherited mutation data for medical research, genetic diagnosis and next-generation sequencing studies. Hum Genet 2017;136(6):665–77.
54. Lek M, Karczewski KJ, Minikel EV, et al. Analysis of protein-coding genetic variation in 60,706 humans. Nature 2016;536:285–91.
55. Benjamini Y, Speed TP. Summarizing and correcting the GC content bias in high-throughput sequencing. Nucleic Acids Res 2012;40(10):e72.
56. Saunders CJ, Miller NA, Soden SE, et al. Rapid whole-genome sequencing for genetic disease diagnosis in neonatal intensive care units. Sci Transl Med 2012;4(154):154ra135.
57. Bamshad MJ, Ng SB, Bigham AW, et al. Exome sequencing as a tool for Mendelian disease gene discovery. Nat Rev Genet 2011;12:745–55.
58. Longoni M, High FA, Qi H, et al. Genome-wide enrichment of damaging de novo variants in patients with isolated and complex congenital diaphragmatic hernia. Hum Genet 2017;136(6):679–91.
59. Horn R, Parker M. Opening Pandora's box?: ethical issues in prenatal whole genome and exome sequencing. Prenat Diagn 2017. https://doi.org/10.1002/pd.5114.
60. Bunnik EM, de Jong A, Nijsingh N, et al. The new genetics and informed consent: differentiating choice to preserve autonomy. Bioethics 2013;27(6):348–55.
61. Pinxten W, Howard HC. Ethical issues raised by whole genome sequencing. Best Pract Res Clin Gastroenterol 2014;28(2):269–79.
62. Gymrek M, McGuire AL, Golan D, et al. Identifying personal genomes by surname inference. Science 2013;339:321–4.

63. Botkin JR, Belmont JW, Berg JS, et al. Points to consider: ethical, legal and psychosocial implications of genetic testing in children and adolescents. Am J Hum Genet 2015;97:6–21.
64. Lacey S, Chung JY, Lin H. A comparison of whole genome sequencing with exome sequencing for family-based association studies. BMC Proc 2014; 8(Suppl 1 Genetic Analysis Workshop 18Vanessa Olmo):S3.
65. Committee opinion no. 640: cell-free DNA screening for fetal aneuploidy. Obstet Gynecol 2015;126(3):e31–7.
66. Fan HC, Gu W, Wang J, et al. Non-invasive prenatal measurement of the fetal genome. Nature 2012;487(7407):320–4.
67. Kitzman JO, Snyder MW, Ventura M, et al. Noninvasive whole-genome sequencing of a human fetus. Sci Transl Med 2012;4(137):137ra76.
68. Bi W, Breman A, Shaw CA, et al. Detection of $\geq$1Mb microdeletions and microduplications in a single cell using custom oligonucleotide arrays. Prenat Diagn 2012;32(1):10–20.
69. Breman AM, Chow JC, U'Ren L, et al. Evidence for feasibility of fetal trophoblastic cell-based noninvasive prenatal testing. Prenat Diagn 2016;36(11):1009–19.

Ethnicity-Based Carrier Screening

Jennifer R. King, MD, MS, Susan Klugman, MD*

KEYWORDS

- Ethnicity • Carrier screening • Autosomal recessive • Preconception

KEY POINTS

- Ethnicity-based carrier screening is an important component of preconception and prenatal care.
- Pretest and posttest counseling are essential to ensure patient understanding.
- Providers should understand the benefits and limitations of the screening tests they offer.
- Expanded carrier screening may replace ethnicity-based carrier screening in the near future.

INTRODUCTION

Ethnicity-based carrier screening for single-gene disorders has been in clinical practice since the 1960s and has expanded over the decades with advancing technology. It has been almost 50 years since Wilson and Jungner[1] published their classic report on the principles and practice of screening for disease. The original criteria established by Wilson and Jungner[1] (**Box 1**) were updated by the World Health Organization in 2008.[2] Important consideration has also been given to applying the modern criteria to the prenatal setting[3,4] (**Box 2**). Understanding the basis for these criteria has become particularly valuable as technology such as whole-exome sequencing and whole-genome sequencing become more common in Western medicine.

Historically, the need for ethnicity-based carrier screening was a result of the recognition of the founder effect, which was first described by Ernst Mayr[5,6] in 1942. A founder effect accounts for the presence of a disease-associated allele at an unusually high frequency in an isolated population. A founder effect can result from the establishment of a new population from a few individuals derived from a

Disclosure: The authors have no financial conflicts or disclosures.
Department of Obstetrics & Gynecology and Women's Health, Division of Reproductive and Medical Genetics, Albert Einstein College of Medicine, Montefiore Medical Center, 1695 East-chester Road, Suite 301, Bronx, NY 10461, USA
* Corresponding author.
E-mail address: sklugman@montefiore.org

Obstet Gynecol Clin N Am 45 (2018) 83–101
https://doi.org/10.1016/j.ogc.2017.10.010
0889-8545/18/© 2017 Elsevier Inc. All rights reserved.

obgyn.theclinics.com

Box 1
Wilson and Jungner[1] carrier screening criteria

1. The condition sought should be an important health problem.

2. There should be an accepted treatment of patients with recognized disease.

3. Facilities for diagnosis and treatment should be available.

4. There should be a recognizable latent or early symptomatic stage.

5. There should be a suitable test or examination.

6. The test should be acceptable to the population.

7. The natural history of the condition, including development from latent to declared disease, should be adequately understood.

8. There should be an agreed-on policy on whom to treat as patients.

9. The cost of case finding (including diagnosis and treatment of patients diagnosed) should be economically balanced in relation to possible expenditure on medical care as a whole.

10. Case finding should be a continuing process and not a once-and-for-all project.

From Wilson JMG, Jungner G. Principles and practice of screening for disease. Geneva (Switzerland): World Health Organization (WHO); 1968; with permission.

---

larger population or from a dramatic reduction in population size followed by rapid expansion, also described as a genetic bottleneck.[7] For example, complete genome sequencing data from 128 Ashkenazi Jewish controls support a narrow population bottleneck of just a few hundred individuals.[8] This narrow bottleneck explains the highly specific genetic variation within the Ashkenazi Jews, despite the current large size of the population. Another term used to account for specific disease-associated alleles found in certain populations is called heterozygote advantage.[9,10] Heterozygote advantage is the favored explanation for descendants from the Mediterranean, southeast Asia (including the Indian subcontinent), the Middle East, and Africa being carriers for hemoglobinopathies. In the past, hemoglobinopathies were found in the geographic regions of malaria endemicity because carriers have some degree of protection against infection.[11,12] Despite this explanation, the net result is a population at increased risk for autosomal recessive diseases.

Box 2
Modern criteria for prenatal carrier screening

1. The natural history of the disorder should be well understood and should severely impair the health of an affected offspring.

2. There should be a high frequency of carriers in the screened population.

3. Technically valid screening methods should be available.

4. The genotypic and phenotypic correlations should be predictable and strong.

5. Prenatal diagnosis and intervention should be valid reproductive options.

Data from Ram KT, Klugman SD. Best practices: antenatal screening for common genetic conditions other than aneuploidy. Curr Opin Obstet Gynecol 2010;22(2):139–45.

Offering ethnicity-based carrier screening is an important component of preconception and prenatal care. Obtaining a family history of the person (and the person's partner, if possible) and establishing ethnicity is essential to determine their inherited risk. Traditionally, ethnic and family background has guided decision making regarding focused population screening. More recently, with the admixture of marriages, pan-ethnic screening for hundreds of disorders has gained in popularity.[13,14] This topic is discussed in Anthony R. Gregg's article, "Expanded Carrier Screening," in this issue.

Timing of carrier screening is always an important consideration. The preferred approach is to perform carrier screening before pregnancy.[15] However, sometimes reimbursement is only available during pregnancy. If that is the case, screening early in pregnancy is best to allow for possible partner screening thereafter and prenatal diagnosis. Concurrent testing of both parents should be considered if timing of the results is critical.

Interpretation of the carrier screening results and posttest genetic counseling are equally significant to the process. If both parents are determined to be carriers for the same autosomal recessive disorder, there is a 25% risk that their offspring will be affected with the disease. If they have the same mutation, the affected offspring would be a homozygote. If they have different mutations in the same gene, the affected offspring with both mutations would be considered a compound heterozygote. During pregnancy, prenatal diagnosis may be pursued after genetic counseling with amniocentesis or chorionic villus sampling. If the disease is confirmed on prenatal diagnostic testing, parents should be offered additional genetic counseling and discussion of the reproductive options. The parents may also decline prenatal diagnostic testing and undergo expectant management until after birth. Carriers should be encouraged to share the information with their relatives. Negative carrier screening results are reassuring but still require genetic counseling. Although the risk of affected offspring is low with negative carrier screening results, the risk is not zero. A residual risk remains that depends on the test performance in the population of the individual being screened. In addition, parents should understand that prenatal carrier screening does not replace newborn screening, and newborn screening should still be conducted at birth.

Preconception carrier screening allows for reproductive options such as in vitro fertilization with preimplantation genetic diagnosis in families in which both parents are known carriers (ie, carrier couples). This technique allows the parents to minimize the risk of an affected offspring but may have other risks.

Carrier frequencies are estimates obtained using disease incidence and the Hardy-Weinberg equation, because the entire population is not screened. In addition, many of these estimates are based on mutation analysis and several laboratories are using sequencing, which may decrease residual risks. The Hardy-Weinberg law states that allele and genotype frequencies in a population remain constant from generation to generation.[16] However, it is also important to note that disease incidence may not follow traditional Hardy-Weinberg equilibrium because affected fetuses may not make it to term.

There are several diseases for which carrier screening has been recommended for the general population by professional organizations. In the United States, the American College of Obstetrics and Gynecology (ACOG) recommends panethnic screening for cystic fibrosis, and most recently spinal muscular atrophy.[17] ACOG also recommends a complete blood count with red blood cell indices to assess for risk of hemoglobinopathy.[17] Similarly, the American College of Medical Genetics (ACMG) recommends population screening for cystic fibrosis and spinal muscular atrophy. **Table 1** provides a summary of currently available ACOG and ACMG carrier screening guidelines. A detailed discussion of some of these disorders is presented later.

DISORDERS
Hemoglobinopathies

Hemoglobinopathies, such as sickle cell disease and thalassemia, are among the most common single-gene disorders worldwide. Approximately 1.1% of couples worldwide are at risk for having children with a hemoglobin disorder and 2.7 per 1000 conceptions are affected.[18] ACOG recommends universal prenatal screening for hemoglobinopathies.[17] All pregnant women should receive a complete blood count with red blood cell indices to assess risk for hemoglobinopathies.[17] Findings necessitating additional screening with hemoglobin electrophoresis include a hypochromic

Table 1
Summary of current American College of Obstetrics and Gynecology and American College of Medical Genetics screening recommendations

Screening Tests	ACOG	ACMG
Hemoglobinopathies	Screening with CBC with RBC indices offered to all women preconception or prenatally Hemoglobin electrophoresis offered to individuals of African, Mediterranean, Middle Eastern, southeast Asian, or West Indian descent	Not addressed
Ashkenazi Jewish panel	Individuals of Ashkenazi Jewish descent should be offered screening for Tay-Sachs disease, Canavan disease, cystic fibrosis, and familial dysautonomia	Individuals of Ashkenazi Jewish descent should be offered screening for Tay-Sachs disease, Canavan disease, cystic fibrosis, familial dysautonomia, Fanconi anemia group C, Niemann-Pick disease type A, Bloom syndrome, mucolipidosis type IV, and Gaucher disease
Cystic fibrosis	Screening offered to all women preconception or prenatally	Screening with 23-mutation panel offered to all women preconception or prenatally
Spinal muscular atrophy	Screening offered to all women preconception or prenatally	Screening offered to all women preconception or prenatally
Fragile X syndrome	Screening offered to women with family history of fragile X–related disorders or undiagnosed intellectual disability, unexplained premature ovarian insufficiency, or increased FSH level before the age of 40 y	Screening offered to individuals with intellectual disability, developmental delay, or autism; women with a family history of fragile X syndrome or undiagnosed intellectual disability; women experiencing reproductive problems associated with increased FSH level

Abbreviations: CBC, complete blood count; FSH, follicle-stimulating hormone; RBC, red blood cell.
Data from Refs.[17,27,39,42,48]

microcytic anemia (low mean corpuscular hemoglobin level and low mean corpuscular volume). Hemoglobin electrophoresis should be obtained in addition to complete blood count in individuals of African, Mediterranean, Middle Eastern, southeast Asian, or West Indian descent. A general approach to screening for hemoglobinopathies is presented in **Fig. 1.**

Sickle Cell Disorders

Dr James Herrick first described sickle cell disease more than 100 years ago.[19] His observations of peculiar elongated and sickle-shaped red blood corpuscles in 1910 later led to it being heralded as the first molecular disease.[19,20] Adult hemoglobin is a tetramer and consists of 2 alpha chains and a combination of 2 beta chains

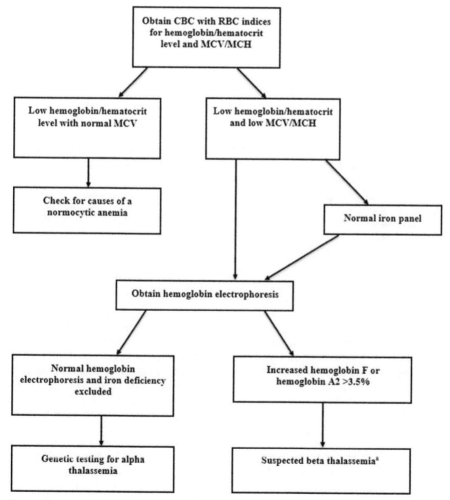

Fig. 1. General approach to screening for thalassemia. [a] Confirm with genetic testing. CBC, complete blood count; RBC, red blood cell; MCH, mean corpuscular hemoglobin; MCV, mean corpuscular volume.

(hemoglobin A [Hb A]), 2 gamma chains (Hb F), or 2 delta chains (Hb A$_2$). The abnormal hemoglobin responsible for sickle cell disease (Hb S) occurs when a single-nucleotide substitution of thymine for adenine occurs in the -globin gene. Heterozygotes of Hb S (Hb AS) are asymptomatic and described as having sickle cell trait, whereas sickle cell anemia occurs in homozygotes of Hb S (Hb SS). This alteration of normal Hb A into Hb S causes a substitution of valine for glutamic acid in the sixth position of the -globin chain, and ultimately a distortion of red blood cell shape under conditions of decreased oxygen tension. The distorted red blood cells increase blood viscosity and can obstruct blood supply within small blood vessels, resulting in painful vaso-occlusive crises within affected organs. These distorted red blood cells are also prone to hemolysis, worsening anemia and decreasing oxygenation further. Affected individuals usually require several blood transfusions over their lifetimes and bone marrow transplants are the only known cure.

Diagnosis of sickle cell disorders is made by hemoglobin electrophoresis. Homozygotes have nearly all their hemoglobin as Hb S, with small amounts of Hb A$_2$ and Hb F. Heterozygotes or those with sickle cell trait can be identified by a larger percentage of Hb A. It is important to identify and properly inform individuals with sickle cell trait because they are at risk for having children with sickle cell disease if their partners also have sickle cell trait. Data from state newborn screening programs in 2010 showed that 1.5% of all infants screened had sickle cell trait.[21] The incidence of sickle cell trait varies among different races and ethnicities; African American infants have the highest incidence at 73.1 cases per 1000 births, compared with 6.9 per 1000 Hispanic infants, 3 per 1000 white infants, and 2.2 per 1000 Asian or Pacific Islander.[21] With appropriate genetic counseling, parents who are both carriers for sickle cell trait may pursue reproductive options such as preimplantation genetic diagnosis or prenatal diagnosis with amniocentesis or chorionic villus sampling.

There are more than 1000 other hemoglobin variants of varying severity that have been discovered.[22] These variants, such as Hb C or Hb E, are rare individually but common collectively and may have important clinical consequences, especially when occurring in combination.[22]

α-Thalassemia

α-Thalassemia carrier status occurs when there is a gene deletion of 2 or more copies of the 4 genes.[23] The severity of the disorder in an affected offspring is correlated with the number of deleted copies of the 4 genes inherited from both parents. Hb H disease results from a deletion of 3 out of 4 genes and is associated with mild to moderate hemolytic anemia. Hemoglobin Bart disease, also called α-thalassemia major, results from the loss of all 4 genes. α-Thalassemia minor (α-thalassemia trait) is caused by deletion of 2 of the genes and results in a mild asymptomatic microcytic anemia. If the deletions are on the same chromosome, they are said to be in cis (−−/) whereas if there is 1 deletion on each chromosome, they are said to be in trans (−/−). Deletion of only 1 of the genes (−/) is clinically unrecognizable and is not detected on standard laboratory testing. These individuals are called silent carriers.

Differences in genotype have important reproductive implications. α-Thalassemia minor is common among persons of Mediterranean, African, West Indian, and southeast Asian descent. In contrast with individuals of African descent, who usually carry their gene deletions in trans (−/−) presentation, individuals with southeast Asian ancestry more commonly carry their gene deletions in cis (−−/) presentation and are at increased risk for hemoglobin H or hemoglobin Bart disease. Individuals with α-thalassemia do not produce any functional alpha globin and therefore cannot form Hb A, F, or A2. α-Thalassemia major is associated with fetal hydrops, intrauterine demise, and preeclampsia.[23] α-Thalassemia trait carriers of African origin do not typically develop fetal hemoglobin Bart disease during pregnancy. Classification and characteristics of α-thalassemia are listed in Table 3 in Carrier Screening for Genetic Conditions, Committee opinion no. 691 by the American College of Obstetricians and Gynecologists.[17]

Occasionally, α-thalassemia may occur as a result of a point mutation resulting in gene malfunction. For example, hemoglobin Constant Spring is an unusual form of silent carrier that is named after the region of Jamaica in which it was discovered and causes no health problems. However, homozygous Constant Spring results in anemia similar to Hb H disease. In addition, the combination of Hb H Constant Spring (when 1 parent is a carrier of α-thalassemia trait and the other is a Constant Spring carrier) results in a more severe anemia than Hb H. α-Thalassemia can also be inherited in combination with sickle cell disease or trait. Both sickle cell trait and sickle cell disease, which affect the chain, can join with heterozygous or homozygous α-thalassemia. In contrast, with Hb H Constant Spring, coinheritance of α-thalassemia decreases the proportion of Hb S and lessens the severity of the hemolytic anemia.[24]

Definitive diagnosis of α-thalassemia is different than the other hemoglobinopathies because it requires direct sequencing DNA analysis of the globin genes. However, the decision to consider DNA analysis usually follows the finding of hypochromic microcytic red blood cells in the setting of a normal Hb A_2 level on hemoglobin electrophoresis (Hb A_2 levels are increased in β-thalassemia). Genetic testing with direct sequencing DNA analysis identifies the number of genes deleted or mutated and whether they are in cis or trans.

Changing patterns of immigration have altered the prevalence of individuals with hemoglobinopathies, particularly thalassemia. Worldwide, the estimated prevalence of the population carrying α-thalassemia was 20.7% in 2008.[18] Southeast Asians and Africans had the highest prevalence, at 44.6% and 41.2%, respectively.[18] With increasing population migration, combinations of the various hemoglobinopathies and thalassemias are expected to increase, presenting new challenges in genetic counseling and prenatal diagnosis.

β-Thalassemia

β-Thalassemia is caused by a mutation in 1 or both beta globin genes, resulting in deficient or absent production of beta chain. The beta chain is necessary for production of Hb A. Individuals who are homozygous have β-thalassemia major (Cooley anemia) or thalassemia intermedia, whereas heterozygotes have β-thalassemia minor. β-Thalassemia major is characterized by severe anemia with resultant extramedullary erythropoiesis; poor growth; and, if left untreated, death within the first decade of life. Treatment is periodic blood transfusions, iron chelation therapy, or bone marrow transplant. Thalassemia intermedia refers to homozygotes with less severe mutations, who have variable amounts of beta chains produced and therefore some Hb A synthesis and a milder anemia. β-Thalassemia minor has a variable amount of beta-chain production and is usually associated with a mild asymptomatic anemia.

β-Thalassemia minor can also occur in combination with Hb S. Affected individuals inherit 1 mutated gene from each parent with the resulting expression of Hb S/thalassemia determined by the type of β-thalassemia mutation and therefore amount of beta globin present. The most severe form has no normal beta-chain pro-duction and therefore no synthesis of Hb A. The resulting severe phenotype, sickle cell-^{0} thalassemia, is similar to homozygous sickle cell disease and occurs more commonly in the Greek, Middle Eastern, and Mediterranean regions. Classification and characteristics of β-thalassemia are listed in **Table 2**.

The world incidence of β-thalassemia is 1:100,000, but the carrier frequency is up to 1 in 7 in high-risk populations.[25,26] Diagnosis of suspected β-thalassemia should be confirmed on hemoglobin electrophoresis. Hb A is severely reduced or absent and increased hemoglobin F and Hb A_2 levels (>3.5%) are present.

Ashkenazi Jewish Genetic Disorders

Ashkenazi Jewish genetic disorders refers to a group of autosomal recessive dis-eases that, although rare in the general population, have an increased frequency in Ashkenazi Jews, notably Jews from Central Europe and eastern Europe. When testing was performed on 9 disorders, it was estimated that between 1 in 4 and 1 in 5 Ashkenazi Jews carry a mutation for one of these disorders.[27] More recent re-ports include testing on a larger number of disorders and estimate this number to be closer to 1 in 3, even 1 in 2.[28,29]

Although extensive panels for screening for Jewish genetic disorders exist, both ACOG and ACMG have specific recommendations regarding which disorders should be screened for. ACOG recommends that carrier screening should be offered for Tay-Sachs disease, Canavan disease, cystic fibrosis, and familial dysautonomia.[17] ACMG recommends screening for the same 4 disorders with the addition of Fanconi anemia group C, Niemann-Pick disease type A, Bloom syndrome, mucolipidosis type IV, and Gaucher disease.[27] ACOG acknowledges that some experts advocate for more comprehensive screening in individuals of Ashkenazi Jewish descent.[17] ACOG recommends additional screening should be considered for Bloom syn-drome, familial hyperinsulinemia, Fanconi anemia, Gaucher disease, glycogen stor-age disease type I, Joubert syndrome, maple syrup urine disease, mucolipidosis type IV, Niemann-Pick disease, and Usher syndrome.[17] ACMG has also published a policy statement including criteria for a particular disorder to be included in pre-conception/prenatal carrier screening.[30] For each disorder included in the panel, the ACMG criteria include that the causative genes, mutations, and mutation fre-quencies should be known in the population being tested, so that a meaningful re-sidual risk in individuals who test negative can be assessed.[30] The ACMG also recommends that disorders should be of a nature such that most at-risk patients

Table 2
Hemoglobin patterns of beta thalassemia

Hemoglobin Type	Normal	Affected		Carrier
		β^0 - Thal Homozygotes (Major)	β$^+$ - Thal Homozygotes or β$^+$/β^0 Compound Heterozygotes (Intermedia)	β - Thal Heterozygotes (Minor)
HbA	96%–98%	0	10%–30%	92%–95%
HbF	<1%	95%–98%	70%–90%	0.5%–4%
HbA$_2$	2%–3%	2%–5%	2%–5%	>3.5%

Data from Telen MJ, Kaufman RE. The mature erythrocyte. In: Lee GR, Paraskevas F, Foerster J, Lukens J, eds. Wintrobe's Clinical Hematology. 10th edition. Baltimore (MD): Lippincott Williams & Wilkins; 1999. p. 207.

and their partners identified would consider having a prenatal diagnosis to facilitate making decisions surrounding reproduction.[30] Carrier frequency, detection rates, and residual risk for the 9 ACMG-recommended Ashkenazi Jewish genetic diseases are listed in **Table 3**.

Tay-Sachs Disease

Tay-Sachs disease is a lysosomal storage disease caused by a deficiency in the enzyme hexosaminidase A. The disease is characterized by a progressive and rapid neurologic deterioration within the first year of life. There is no treatment and the maximum life expectancy is 5 years. The carrier frequency is 1 in 30 in the Ashkenazi Jewish population, compared with 1:300 in non-Jewish individuals.[17] The carrier frequency of Tay-Sachs disease is also increased relative to the general population in individuals of French Canadian and Cajun descent at ∼1 in 50.[17] Both ACOG and ACMG recommend carrier screening in. these populations as well. In the future, Tay-Sachs screening may become panethnic because children with Tay-Sachs who are born now are often not Ashkenazi Jewish.[31] There are several reports indicating the possibility of mutations in the Irish population and other non-Ashkenazi Jewish European populations; however, studies are ongoing.[32,33]

There are 2 forms of screening available: enzyme analysis and DNA analysis via mutation analysis. Enzyme assays directly measure hexosaminidase A and hexosaminidase B levels in serum, leukocytes, and platelets. Carriers have decreased hexosaminidase A activity or increased activity of hexosaminidase B. Enzyme analysis can

Table 3
Characteristics of Ashkenazi Jewish genetic diseases (American College of Medical Genetics recommended for screening)

Disease	Carrier Frequency	Type of Test	Detection Rate (%)	Residual Risk After Negative Result
Tay-Sachs disease	1 in 30	DNA analysis or enzyme assay	92–99	1:484-1:1451
Canavan disease	1 in 41	DNA mutation analysis	97	1:2000
Cystic fibrosis	1 in 24	DNA mutation analysis	94	1:1000
Familial dysautonomia	1 in 32	DNA mutation analysis	98	1:3101
Fanconi anemia group C	1 in 89	DNA mutation analysis	99	1:8801
Niemann-Pick disease type A	1 in 90	DNA mutation analysis	97	1:1781
Bloom syndrome	1 in 107	DNA mutation analysis	99	1:1981–1:3301
Mucolipidosis type IV	1 in 127	DNA mutation analysis	95	1:2521
Gaucher disease	1 in 18	DNA mutation analysis	95	1:281

Data from Carrier Screening for Genetic Conditions. Committee opinion no. 691. American College of Obstetricians and Gynecologists. Obstet Gynecol 2017;129(3):e41–55; and Gross SJ, Pletcher BA, Monaghan KG. Carrier screening in individuals of Ashkenazi Jewish descent. Genet Med 2008;10(1):54–6.

also be performed on amniocytes or chorionic villus cells. However, serum enzyme levels can be unreliable in pregnancy and in women on hormonal contraception, creating false increases and increasing the likelihood of a false-negative screen. Therefore, leukocyte or platelet screening must be used in women who are pregnant or using oral contraception.[34] When screening in pregnancy with DNA analysis, a detection rate of 92% to 99% is noted with the 3 most common mutations.[27] In a carrier screening program with this detection rate, 95% of affected fetuses can be detected.[34] However, 1 study noted that many carriers can be missed if mutation analysis is used without enzyme testing.[35] It has yet to be determined whether enzyme analysis will still play an important role when sequencing is used for carrier screening in the Ashkenazi Jewish population, although it has been explored in the non–Ashkenazi Jewish population.[36]

Canavan Disease

Canavan disease is a neurodegenerative leukodystrophy caused by a deficiency of the enzyme aspartoacylase, which leads to increased N-acetylaspartic acid levels in the brain and urine. Disease onset is in the first few months of life and it is usually fatal within the first few years of life. The carrier frequency is 1 in 41 in the Ashkenazi Jewish population.[27] Mutation analysis for the 2 most common mutations in the Ashkenazi Jewish population detects 97.4% of carriers.[27] Although an enzyme assay exists, it cannot be performed on amniocytes, chorionic villi cells, or blood because of normally low activity levels in these tissues. Therefore, if prenatal diagnosis is desired and the parental mutations cannot be identified, the ACMG recommends amniocentesis to measure the concentration of N-acetylaspartic acid levels in the amniotic fluid.[34] If a prenatal procedure is performed, the detection rate would be ~95% for affected fetuses.[34]

Cystic Fibrosis

Cystic fibrosis is discussed in more detail elsewhere. In the Ashkenazi Jewish population, the carrier frequency is 1 in 24.[17] Mutation analysis for 5 mutations identifies 94% of carriers in this population.[34]

Familial Dysautonomia

Familial dysautonomia is a progressive sensorimotor neuropathy with severe, life-threatening crises resulting from sympathetic autonomic dysfunction. Nearly all cases of familial dysautonomia occur in the Ashkenazi Jewish population, with a carrier frequency of 1 in 32.[17] One mutation accounts for more than 98% of the mutations in the Ashkenazi Jewish population.[27] A second mutation accounts for the remainder of the known mutations. Screening for these 2 mutations via DNA mutation analysis provides a detection rate of more than 99%.[27] At this detection rate, at least 99% of affected fetuses can be detected with a prenatal diagnostic testing.[34]

Fanconi Anemia Group C

Fanconi anemia is associated with congenital anomalies, progressive bone marrow failure, and a higher prevalence of hematologic malignancies and solid tumors caused by disruption of normal DNA repair. Age of onset varies from birth to 9 years and median survival ranges from 16 to 23 years. The carrier frequency is 1 in 89 in the Ashkenazi Jewish population.[27] A single mutation is responsible for most of the disease in Ashkenazi Jews and DNA testing identifies more than 99% of carriers.[27]

With prenatal diagnostic testing, more than 98% of affected fetuses can be detected.[34]

Niemann-Pick Disease Type A

Niemann-Pick disease is a lysosomal storage disorder caused by a deficiency of acid sphingomyelinase. Disease onset is within the first few months of life and rapid neurologic deterioration leads to death in early childhood. The carrier frequency is 1 in 90 in the Ashkenazi Jewish population.[27] Screening for the 3 common mutations identified provides a carrier detection rate of 97% and a detection rate for an affected fetus of 94% with prenatal diagnostic testing.[34]

Bloom Syndrome

Bloom syndrome is a chromosome instability disorder characterized by growth delays, intellectual impairment, immunodeficiency, and cancer predisposition. Clinical features are attributed to increased chromosome breakage and sister chromatid exchange. The mean age of death is 28 years, usually caused by cancer of hematologic or gastrointestinal origin. The carrier frequency is 1 in 107 in the Ashkenazi Jewish population.[27] A complex frameshift mutation accounts for almost all patients with Bloom syndrome. Testing via DNA mutation analysis detects more than 99% of carriers.[27] Similarly, prenatal diagnostic testing detects at least 99% of affected fetuses.[34]

Mucolipidosis Type IV

Mucolipidosis type IV is a lysosomal storage disease characterized by growth and developmental delays, severe intellectual disability, and ophthalmologic abnormalities. Although affected individuals may have a normal life expectancy, most are diagnosed by the age of 2 years and never attain language skills or motor function beyond that age. The carrier frequency is 1 in 127.[27] Carrier screening for the 2 associated mutations provides a detection rate of 95% in the Ashkenazi Jewish population.[27] At this detection rate, approximately 90% of affected fetuses can be detected with amniocentesis or chorionic villus sampling.[34]

Gaucher Disease

Gaucher disease is a lysosomal storage disease caused by a deficiency in the enzyme glucocerebrosidase. The disease is subdivided into 3 types, with type 1 the most common in Ashkenazi Jews. The disease is characterized by thrombocytopenia, hepatosplenomegaly, and bone fractures. Although onset may occur in infancy, half of patients do not present until after 45 years of age and some cases are mild or asymptomatic. The median life expectancy is 68 years. Gaucher disease is considered the most prevalent genetic disorder among Ashkenazi Jews, with a carrier frequency of 1 in 18.[27] More than 200 mutant alleles responsible for Gaucher disease have been identified but 4 contribute to most of the disease in the Ashkenazi Jewish population. Targeted DNA analysis for the 4 most common mutations detects up to 94.6% of carriers.[27] At a carrier detection rate of 95%, the detection rate for affected fetuses with prenatal diagnostic procedures is approximately 90%.[34] Enzyme activity assays can also help detect carriers who do not have one of the common mutations. The addition of enzyme activity can increase the testing sensitivity in the Ashkenazi Jewish population. Enzyme activity testing can also be used for prenatal diagnosis on cells obtained by amniocentesis or chorionic villus sampling in parents identified as carriers but without a known mutation. However, counseling parents of an affected fetus is difficult given the wide variability in phenotypic expression and the availability of enzyme-replacement therapy. Routine carrier screening for Gaucher disease is controversial and requires proper genetic counseling. In addition, Gaucher disease carriers are at a slightly increased risk of developing Parkinson disease later in life, which is important to discuss with individuals undergoing carrier testing.[37]

Cystic Fibrosis

Both ACOG and ACMG recommend cystic fibrosis carrier screening for all women in the preconception period or during pregnancy. Cystic fibrosis is a pulmonary and exocrine pancreatic disease characterized by chronic lung disease, recurrent pneumonia, pancreatic insufficiency, malabsorption, and diabetes mellitus. The average life expectancy is 42 years with respiratory failure the most common cause of death. The disease is the most common life-threatening autosomal recessive condition in the non-Hispanic white population, with a disease incidence of 1 in 2500 and a carrier frequency of 1 in 25.[17] Carrier frequencies for other races or ethnic groups are listed in **Table 1**. Because of difficulty in assigning a single ethnicity to individuals, in 2005 ACOG recommended all women be offered cystic fibrosis carrier screening.[17]

Cystic fibrosis is caused by mutations in the cystic fibrosis transmembrane regulator gene. More than 2000 mutations have been identified,[38] but current guidelines from ACMG recommend use of a standard panel including the 23 most common mutations, at a minimum.[39] Detection rates vary depending on the race or ethnic group (**Table 4**). Expanded panels may be appropriate for those with lower detection rates using the standard 23-mutation panel. Although DNA sequencing of the complete CFTR gene is not recommended for routine carrier screening, it may be considered under certain circumstances. Individuals with a negative carrier screen but a personal or family history of cystic fibrosis, newborns with a positive screening result but negative standard mutation panel, or male individuals with congenital bilateral absence of the vas deferens may be candidates for CFTR gene sequencing.[17] If parents are found to be carriers, prenatal diagnostic testing can be performed via chorionic villus sampling or amniocentesis.

Spinal Muscular Atrophy

Spinal muscular atrophy is a neurodegenerative disease resulting in progressive muscular atrophy and paralysis. The disease has several subtypes based on age of onset and clinical course. New gene-replacement therapies have resulted in longer

Table 4
Cystic fibrosis detection and carrier risk among different races and ethnic groups

Racial or Ethnic Group	Detection Rate (%)	Carrier Frequency	Residual Risk
Ashkenazi Jewish	94	1 in 24	1:380
Non-Hispanic white	88	1 in 25	1:200
Hispanic white	72	1 in 58	1:200
African American	64	1 in 61	1:170
Asian American	49	1 in 94	1:180

Detection rate based on 23-mutation panel.
From American College of Medical Genetics and Genomics. Technical standards and guidelines for CFTR mutation testing. American College of Medical Genetics Standards and Guidelines for Clinical Genetics Laboratories. Bethesda (MD): ACMG; 2011. Available at: http://www.acmg.net/docs/CFTR_Mutation_Testing_2011.pdf. Retrieved September 12, 2016; with permission.

survival and better motor function.[40,41] However there is no cure. Type I (Werdnig-Hoffman) is the most severe, with onset before 6 months of age and is usually fatal by 2 years of age because of respiratory failure. Type II is the most common and is of intermediate severity. Onset is typically before 2 years of age, with respiratory failure and death frequently occurring during adolescence. Type III (Kugelberg-Welander) is the least severe, presenting after 18 months of age with variable muscular weakness. Affected individuals usually reach all major motor milestones and many are able to ambulate without assistance and have normal life expectancies. Two additional sub-types are type IV, which has adult onset, and type O, which develops prenatally.

Spinal muscular atrophy is the second most common lethal autosomal recessive condition in white people, with a disease incidence of 1 in 6000 to 1,10,000, and is reported to be the leading genetic cause of infant death.[17] However, until 2017, only ACMG recommended population screening for spinal muscular atrophy.[42] ACOG previously recommended screening only those with a family history of spinal muscular atrophy or spinal muscular atrophy–like disease, or those without a family history who request it and receive genetic counseling regarding test limitations.[43] Recently, ACOG aligned with ACMG and recommended panethnic screening to all women considering pregnancy or currently pregnant after appropriate genetic counseling.[17]

Identification of spinal muscular atrophy carriers can be complicated. There are 2 survival motor neuron (SMN) genes associated with spinal muscular atrophy: SMN1 and SMN2. SMN1 is considered the active gene with a homozygous deletion in both copies occurring in more than 95% of affected individuals. Variable gene copies of SMN2 (0–3) can exist on each chromosome and seem to modify the disease. A higher number of SMN2 copies are correlated with milder disease, although SMN2 copy number cannot predict phenotype. Carrier testing requires a quantitative assay that provides the SMN1 copy number, with detection of a single normal copy of SMN1 indicating a carrier state. This gene dosage assay is useful when there is 1 SMN1 gene on each chromosome (a trans configuration). However, 3% to 4% of the general population has 2 copies of SMN1 on 1 chromosome and no copies on the other (a cis configuration).[17] These individuals cannot be detected as carriers via gene dosage analysis even though 1 of their chromosomes lacks the SMN1 gene. African Americans, specifically, are more likely to have their SMN1 genes in cis configuration. Gene dosage analysis has a detection rate of 71% in African Americans, compared with more than 90% in other ethnic groups.[17] Therefore, genetic counseling should include a discussion of the residual risk, particularly when gene dosage assay results are negative. Detection rates, carrier frequency, and residual risk by racial or ethnic

Table 5
Spinal muscular atrophy detection and carrier risk among different races and ethnic groups

Racial or Ethnic Group	Detection Rate (%)	Carrier Frequency	Residual Risk with 2 Copies SMN1	Residual Risk with 3 Copies SMN1
White	95	1 in 35	1:632	1:3500
Ashkenazi Jewish	90	1 in 41	1:350	1:4000
Asian	93	1 in 53	1:628	1:5000
African American	71	1 in 66	1:121	1:3000
Hispanic	91	1 in 117	1:1061	1:11,000

From Hendrickson BC, Donohoe C, Akmaev VR, et al. Differences in SMN1 allele frequencies among ethnic groups within North America. J Med Genet 2009;46:641–4; with permission.

group are provided in **Table 5**. The residual risk to be a spinal muscular atrophy carrier can be decreased by specific single nucleotide polymorphism testing offered by some laboratories, therefore decreasing the concerns regarding cis configuration and improving overall detection rates.[44]

Fragile X Syndrome

Fragile X syndrome is the most common cause of inherited intellectual disability and is found in all ethnic groups. The incidence is 1 in 3600 boys and 1 in 4000 to 6000 girls, with a carrier frequency of 1 in 257 for women without known risk factors.[45] Intellectual disability can range from learning disabilities to more severe cognitive and behavioral disabilities, including autism spectrum disorders and attention-deficit/hyperactivity disorder. Other characteristic features include long narrow face with prominent ears, enlarged testes, joint laxity, hypotonia, and delay in speech and motor skills. Boys typically show significant intellectual disability, whereas/girls tend to have more mild intellectual impairment and variable physical features.

Fragile X syndrome has X-linked transmission; however, the molecular genetics are complex. The disorder is caused by the expansion of an unstable trinucleotide repeat on the fragile X mental retardation 1 (FMR1) gene, which is usually accompanied by abnormal hypermethylation and gene silencing. The number of trinucleotide repeats classifies the form of the disease: unaffected (<45), intermediate or gray zone (45–54), premutation (55–200), full mutation (>200) (**Table 6**). Expansion of a premutation to a full mutation occurs almost exclusively from female carriers; male carrier transmission is rare. Risk of expansion increases with increasing size of the premutation, such that, when the maternal number of repeats is more than 100, risk of expansion to full mutation is 98%.[17] Mosaicism can be present both with repeat size and methylation and generally results in a lesser intellectual disability than completely methylated full mutations.

Premutation carriers have a phenotype that is distinct from fragile X syndrome. Male patients who carry the premutation are at increased risk for a tremor and ataxia disorder (fragile X–associated tremor/ataxia syndrome [FXTAS]). Female patients, to a lesser extent, are at increased risk of FXTAS, as well as premature ovarian failure.

Table 6
Fragile X syndrome mutation status and expansion risk

Maternal Number of Triplet Repeats	Mutation Status	Risk of Expansion to Full Mutation (%)
<45	Unaffected	—
45–54	Intermediate	—
55–59	Premutation	4
60–69	Premutation	5
70–79	Premutation	31
80–89	Premutation	58
90–99	Premutation	80
100–200	Premutation	98
>200	Full mutation	100

From Nolin SL, Brown WT, Glicksman A, et al. Expansion of the fragile X CGG repeat in females with premutation or intermediate alleles. Am J Hum Genet 2003;72:454–64; with permission.

The presence of AGG interrupters within the CGG repeats in premutation carriers has recently been studied and noted to potentially modify the risk of a CGG expansion in offspring.[46,47]

Currently, both ACOG and ACMG recommend a risk-based approach to screening for fragile X syndrome. ACOG recommends offering women considering pregnancy or already pregnant fragile X carrier testing if there is a family history of fragile X–related disorders or undiagnosed intellectual disability.[17] They also recommend offering screening to women with unexplained premature ovarian insufficiency or increased follicle-stimulating hormone levels before the age of 40 years.[17] ACMG makes similar recommendations.[48] The recommended method of screening for fragile X syndrome carriers is via molecular genetic testing. Both polymerase chain reaction (PCR) and Southern blotting can be used for the detection of the FMR1 allele expansions; however, PCR has some limitations. Large repeats may be more difficult to detect by PCR and PCR cannot detect mosaicism or methylation status. Southern blot, although more labor intensive, detects mosaicism and methylation status and should be performed for PCR-detected premutations and full mutations. If a carrier is identified, prenatal diagnostic testing can be performed by amniocentesis. Methylation is not fully established at the time of chorionic villus sampling, therefore amniocentesis is the recommended method for prenatal diagnosis.

DISCUSSION

Population-based screening is an important part of preconception and prenatal care. A detailed family history and racial/ethnic ancestry assist with tailoring screening recommendations to meet the needs of the couple. A summary of risk-based screening recommendations is included in **Fig. 2**.

There are limitations to this approach to carrier screening. Society has become increasingly multiracial and multiethnic. According to the United States Census data, the population reporting multiple races increased by 32% from 2000 to 2010.[49] Data also showed that 10% of households are interracial or interethnic married couples.[49] Unmarried interracial or interethnic couples were almost twice that at 18%.[49] In addition, individuals have increasingly inaccurate knowledge of their ancestry. The subjective nature of self-identification was shown in a study of 1752 individuals from the National Marrow Donor program, which found that nearly 1 in 5 respondents provided inconsistent answers between their reported race/ethnicity and geographic ancestry.[50] Further, it is important to recognize that genetic disorders do not occur exclusively in specific ethnic groups and testing for individual genetic disorders restricts the amount genetic information available to patients. A study of 346,790 individuals who underwent expanded carrier screening showed the limitations of ethnicity-based carrier screening using modeled fetal risk of genetic disease.[51] Data from expanded carrier screening revealed that many racial/ethnic categories have a risk of a profound or severe genetic disease that may not be detected by the guidelines present at the time of the analysis.[51]

Advances in technology are rapidly changing the field of genetics. High-throughput genotyping and sequencing allows carrier testing for hundreds of genetic conditions. In addition, clustered regularly interspaced short palindromic repeats are likely to change the future management of single-gene disorders. A time may be approaching time when population-based carrier screening will be abandoned in favor of expanded carrier screening. However, although expanded carrier screening offers more comprehensive screening, there are challenges to implementing this method. Patient

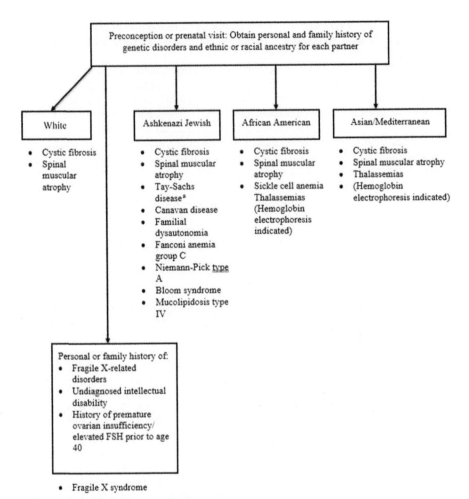

Fig. 2. Summary of population-based carrier screening recommendations. [a] Also screen in individuals of French Canadian or Cajun descent.

management becomes more complex as providers and couples are faced with more unknowns. Before expanded carrier screening can replace population-based screening, providers should understand the risks and benefits.

REFERENCES

1. Wilson JMG, Jungner G. Principles and practice of screening for disease. Geneva, Switzerland: WHO; 1968. Available from: http://www.who.int/bulletin/volumes/86/4/07-050112BP.pdf.
2. Andermann A, Blancquaert I, Beauchamp S, et al. Revisiting Wilson and Jungner in the genomic age: a review of screening criteria over the past 40 years. Bull World Health Organ 2008;86:317–9.
3. Ram KT, Klugman SD. Best practices: antenatal screening for common genetic conditions other than aneuploidy. Curr Opin Obstet Gynecol 2010;22(2):139–45.

4. de Jong A, Dondorp WJ, Frints SG, et al. Advances in prenatal screening: the ethical dimension. Nat Rev Genet 2011;12(9):657–63.
5. Mayr E. Systematics and the origin of species. New York: Columbia University Press; 1942.
6. Bajaj K, Gross SJ. Carrier screening: past, present, and future. J Clin Med 2014; 3(3):1033–42.
7. Amos W, Harwood J. Factors affecting levels of genetic diversity in natural populations. Philos Trans R Soc Lond B Biol Sci 1998;353:177–86.
8. Carmi S, Hui KY, Kochav E, et al. Sequencing an Ashkenazi reference panel supports population-targeted personal genomics and illuminates Jewish and European origins. Nat Commun 2014;5:4835.
9. Haldane JBS. Disease and evolution. La Ricerca Scientifica 1949;19:68–76.
10. Haldane JBS. The rate of mutation of human genes. Hereditas 1949;35(S1): 267–73.
11. Hedrick PW. Population genetics of malaria resistance in humans. Heredity 2011; 107:283–304.
12. Aidoo M, Terlouw DJ, Kolczak MS, et al. Protective effects of the sickle cell gene against malaria morbidity and mortality. Lancet 2002;359(9314):1311–2.
13. van der Hout S, Holtkamp KC, Henneman L, et al. Advantages of expanded universal carrier screening: what is at stake? Eur J Hum Genet 2016;25(1):17–21.
14. Nazareth SB, Lazarin GA, Goldberg JD. Changing trends in carrier screening for genetic disease in the United States. Prenat Diagn 2015;35(10):931–5.
15. Carrier Screening in the Age of Genomic Medicine. Committee opinion no. 690. American College of Obstetricians and Gynecologists. Obstet Gynecol 2017; 129(3):e35–40.
16. Stern C. The Hardy-Weinberg Law. Science 1943;97(2510):137–8.
17. Carrier Screening for Genetic Conditions. Committee opinion no. 691. American College of Obstetricians and Gynecologists. Obstet Gynecol 2017;129(3): e41–55.
18. Modell B, Darlison M. Global epidemiology of haemoglobin disorders and derived service indicators. Bull World Health Organ 2008;86:480–7.
19. Herrick JB. Peculiar elongated and sickle-shaped red blood corpuscles in a case of severe anemia. JAMA 2014;312(10):1063.
20. Steinberg MH. Sickle cell anemia, the first molecular disease: overview of molecular etiology, pathophysiology, and therapeutic approaches. ScientificWorldJournal 2008;8:1295–324.
21. Ojodu J, Hulihan MM, Pope SN, et al. Centers for Disease Control and Prevention (CDC). Incidence of sickle cell trait–United States, 2010. MMWR Morb Mortal Wkly Rep 2014;63(49):1155–8.
22. Thom CS, Dickson CF, Gell DA, et al. Hemoglobin variants: biochemical properties and clinical correlates. Cold Spring Harb Perspect Med 2013;3(3):a011858.
23. ACOG Committee on Obstetrics. ACOG practice bulletin no. 78: hemoglobinopathies in pregnancy. Obstet Gynecol 2007;109(1):229–37.
24. Embury SH, Dozy AM, Miller J, et al. Concurrent sickle-cell anemia and alpha-thalassemia: effect on severity of anemia. N Engl J Med 1982;306(5):270.
25. Galanello R, Origa R. Beta-thalassemia. Orphanet J Rare Dis 2010;5:11.
26. Cousens NE, Gaff CL, Metcalfe SA, et al. Carrier screening for beta-thalassaemia: a review of international practice. Eur J Hum Genet 2010;18(10):1077–83.
27. Gross SJ, Pletcher BA, Monaghan KG. Carrier screening in individuals of Ashkenazi Jewish descent. Genet Med 2008;10(1):54–6.

28. Scott SA, Edelmann L, Liu L, et al. Experience with carrier screening and prenatal diagnosis for 16 Ashkenazi Jewish genetic diseases. Hum Mutat 2010;31(11): 1240–50.

29. Arjunan A, Litwack K, Collins N, et al. Carrier screening in the era of expanding genetic technology. Genet Med 2016;18(12):1214–7.

30. Grody WW, Barry TH, Gregg AR, et al. ACMG position statement on prenatal/preconception expanded carrier screening. Genet Med 2013;15(6):482–3.

31. McGinniss M, Kaback M. Heterozygote testing and carrier screening. In: Rimoin D, Connor M, Pyeritz R, et al, editors. Emery and Rimoin's principles and practice of medical genetics, 1, 5th edition. Philadelphia: Churchill Livingstone; 2007. p. 627–36.

32. Akerman B, Natowicz MR, Kaback M, et al. Novel mutations and DNA-based screening in non-Jewish carriers of Tay-Sachs disease. Am J Hum Genet 1997; 60:1099–106.

33. Branda KJ, Tomczak J, Natowicz MR. Heterozygosity for Tay-Sachs and Sandhoff diseases in non-Jewish Americans with ancestry from Ireland, Great Britain, or Italy. Genet Test 2004;8(2):174–80.

34. Monaghan KG, Feldman GL, Paolmaki GE, et al. Technical standards and guidelines for reproductive screening in the Ashkenazi Jewish population. Genet Med 2008;10(1):57–72.

35. Schneider A, Nakagawa S, Keep R, et al. Population-based Tay-Sachs screening among Ashkenazi Jewish young adults in the 21st century: hexosaminidase A enzyme assay is essential for accurate testing. Am J Med Genet A 2009; 149A(11):2444–7.

36. Mehta N, Lazarin GA, Spiegel E, et al. Tay-Sachs carrier screening by enzyme and molecular analyses in the New York City minority population. Genet Test Mol Biomarkers 2016;20(9):504–9.

37. Sidransky E, Nalls MA, Aasly JO, et al. Multicenter analysis of glucocerebrosidase mutations in Parkinson's disease. N Engl J Med 2009;361:1651–61.

38. Cystic Fibrosis Centre, Hospital for Sick Children. Cystic fibrosis mutation database. Available at: http://www.genet.sickkids.on.ca/StatisticsPage.html. Accessed June 15, 2017.

39. Watson MS, Cutting GR, Desnick RJ, et al. Cystic fibrosis population carrier screening: 2004 revision of American College of Medical Genetics mutation panel. Genet Med 2004;6:387–91.

40. Mendell JR, Al-Zaidy S, Shell R, et al. Single-dose gene-replacement therapy for spinal muscular atrophy. N Engl J Med 2017;37(18):1713–22.

41. Finkel RS, Mercuri E, Darras BT, et al. Nusinersen versus sham control in infantile-onset spinal muscular Atrophy. N Engl J Med 2017;377(18):1723–32.

42. Prior TW. Carrier screening for spinal muscular atrophy. Genet Med 2008;10: 840–2.

43. Spinal muscular atrophy. Committee opinion no. 432. American College of Obstetricians and Gynecologists. Obstet Gynecol 2009;113(5):1194–6.

44. Luo M, Liu L, Peter I, et al. An Ashkenazi Jewish SMN1 haplotype specific to duplication alleles improves pan-ethnic carrier screening for spinal muscular atrophy. Genet Med 2014;16(2):149–56.

45. Cronister A, Teicher J, Rohlfs EM, et al. Prevalence and instability of fragile X alleles: implications for offering fragile X prenatal diagnosis. Obstet Gynecol 2008; 111:596–601.

46. Yrigollen CM, Durbin-Johnson B, Gane L, et al. AGG interruptions within the maternal FMR1 gene reduce the risk of offspring with fragile X syndrome. Genet Med 2012;14(8):729–36.
47. Nolin SL, Sah S, Glicksman A, et al. Fragile X AGG analysis provides new risk predictions for 45-69 repeat alleles. Am J Med Genet A 2013;161A(4):771–8.
48. Sherman S, Pletcher BA, Driscoll DA. Fragile X syndrome: diagnostic and carrier testing. Genet Med 2005;7:584–7.
49. US Census Bureau (2012). Households and families: 2010. Available at: https://www.census.gov/prod/cen2010/briefs/c2010br-14.pdf.
50. Hollenbach JA, Saperstein A, Albrecht M, et al. Race, ethnicity and ancestry in unrelated transplant matching for the national marrow donor program: a comparison of multiple forms of self-identification with genetics. PLoS One 2015;10(8): e0135960.
51. Haque IS, Lazarin GA, Kang HP, et al. Modeled fetal risk of genetic diseases identified by expanded carrier screening. JAMA 2016;316(7):734–42.

Expanded Carrier Screening

Anthony R. Gregg, MD, MBA

KEYWORDS

- Prenatal carrier screening • Expanded carrier screening • Genetic counseling
- Perceptions of Uncertainties in Genome Sequencing (PUGS) scale

KEY POINTS

- The goal of prenatal carrier screening is to provide information to couples considering or with an ongoing pregnancy.
- Couples who select this elective screening have an opportunity to learn whether there is mendelian risk rather than population risk of an affected fetus.
- Couples that select screening have the option of screening for a limited number of conditions, or an expanded number of conditions.
- The Perception of Uncertainties in Genome Sequencing scale offers a framework around which pretest and posttest counseling can be considered.

SCREENING

The term screening is important to understand. Classically, this refers to applying an imperfect test (eg, Papanicolaou smear for cervical cancer) or process (eg, travel questionnaire used during the Ebola epidemic) to identify asymptomatic patients within a population. The imperfection in a screening test refers to the acceptance of false-positive and false-negative results to improve case finding. Carrier screening in genetics attempts to determine, among asymptomatic patients, those capable of passing genes or genetic risk to future generations. This context refers to the population addressed by screening. Prenatal carrier screening is intended to identify asymptomatic, reproductive-aged individuals, so that risk of carrying an affected child can be specified. The target population is couples who are pregnant or planning to become pregnant.[1] There are 2 other dimensions to which the word screening is attached. These dimensions relate to the number of genes (ie, conditions) and the number of genetic variants. The ability to analyze multiple genes and variants simultaneously (with the same sample) set the stage for screening panels. These panels first reflected

Conflict of Interest: The author reports no conflict of interest.
Department of Obstetrics and Gynecology, University of Florida College of Medicine, PO Box 100294, Gainesville, FL 32610-0294, USA
E-mail address: anthonygregg50@gmail.com

genotyping (slow throughput) efforts to return results for more than one gene and variant simultaneously. With current sequencing technology, reported genes and variants are now arbitrary and reflect inconsistent efforts by companies to return results for conditions of interest to society, providers, and their patients. Advances in sequencing technology led to a new term, expanded carrier screening (ECS). In the prenatal setting this expansion allows consideration of panethnic screening, which means the population is not restricted. Expansion also means the number of genes and their variants reported is a function of the laboratories and any restrictions placed on them (eg, time, reimbursement, or regulation). In the clinical setting, ECS has additional implications. Prenatal carrier screening has extended beyond asymptomatic carriers of recessive conditions to include presymptomatic carriers of X-linked and semidominant conditions. The application of screening now has a spectrum and this key concept can be depicted using a Rubik cube (**Fig. 1**).

The Rubik cube matrix has 3 axes. The X axis depicts the populations screened, the Y axis the variants considered in the screening strategy, and the Z axis represents the genes or conditions being evaluated. Red, blue, and green dots denote the magnitude along each axis from highest (red) to lowest (green). The most intensive screening program would be to interrogate an entire population (panethnic; X axis) using sequencing technology (Y axis) and then reporting out information for a large number of genes (Z axis). The least intensive (all green dots on the cube) would be the application of polymerase chain reaction for delta F508 in a family with a proband known to have cystic fibrosis (homozygous delta F508) based on clinical symptoms and prior application of a diagnostic panel. The least intensive application (all green on the cube) is one in which genotyping methods are used for diagnostic purposes. In this case, the risk of affected family members is mendelian in magnitude. When the risk of an asymptomatic carrier moves from population-based (eg, 1/25 for cystic fibrosis) risk to

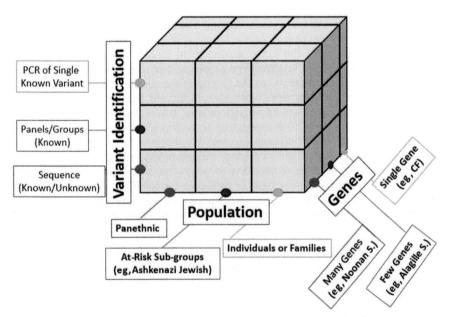

Fig. 1. The Rubik cube model of prenatal diagnosis and carrier screening has 3 axes: population, screened variants, and genes. The red, blue, and green dots indicate stratification across the spectrum. CF, cystic fibrosis; PCR, polymerase chain reaction; S, syndrome.

mendelian (eg, 1/3 for an adult sibling of an affected family member), this moves along the axes of the cube from a screening to a diagnostic paradigm.

HISTORICAL PERSPECTIVE

Genotyping technology available in the early 1990s allowed the molecular diagnosis of conditions characterized by a severe phenotype (eg, cystic fibrosis) within families. At that time the goal was to interrogate a known gene and only a few known pathogenic alleles. High throughput was not a characteristic of these approaches. This process was molecular inquiry for diagnostic purposes. As stated, this utility is represented by the green dots on the Rubik cube axes (see **Fig. 1**). Professional organizations considered the application of genotyping technologies for individual conditions[2,3] and for specific ethnic groups.[4] Prenatal carrier screening used genotyping with the intent of identifying recessive alleles in asymptomatic people. The conditions/genes chosen for screening were enriched in subgroups of the population and were chosen by virtue of the known pathogenic variants, known genes, and severe phenotypes.

Two major scientific accomplishments changed the speed at which screening for mendelian conditions was adopted. Publication of the first complete draft of the human genome sequence[5,6] led the way. The term draft is used to recognize that regions of the genome were/are not fully characterized, which means that a negative screening result always leaves a residual risk (RR; a chance that the patient remains a carrier). RR is calculated as: carrier frequency in a population screened × (1 − detection rate for that population). Over time, sequencing data uncover new pathogenic variants and some pathogenic variants are determined to be nonpathogenic as more clinical information becomes available.[7,8] These changes resulting from new information increase and decrease the detection rate respectively. Furthermore, population carrier frequency varies by ethnicity. In populations characterized as closed with respect to reproduction, fewer pathogenic variants account for a large proportion of disease.[9] For example, in the Ashkenazi Jewish population, 2 pathogenic variants in the HEXA (hexosaminidase A) gene cause more than 90% of the severe disease phenotype. In non–Ashkenazi Jewish, the same 2 variants account for 35% of the severe disease.[10]

Hardy-Weinberg equilibrium can be used to determine the frequency of a phenotype within a population.[11] However, this can only be done under specific conditions (**Box 1, Table 1**). The binomial equation is used when there are 2 possible alleles, p and q. Allele frequency can be determined by counting chromosomes with p or q

Box 1
Hardy-Weinberg equilibrium: criteria
Large population
Random mating
Reproductive fitness is not altered by alleles
No migration to affect allele frequency
No genetic drift to affect allele frequency
Alleles do not undergo mutations
Data from Hardy GH. Mendelian proportions in a mixed population. Science 1908;28(706):49–50.

Table 1	
Hardy-Weinberg equilibrium: equations	
Hardy-Weinberg	$(p + q)^2 = q^2 + 2pq + p^2$
Sum of all alleles	$p + q = 1$
Alleles at a locus (n)	$(p_1 + p_2 + ... p_n)^2$

q may be the frequency of the variant allele or all variant alleles, depending on use of equation.
p is the frequency of the wild-type (normal) allele in the population.
n is the number of alleles possible at a specific locus.
Data from Hardy GH. Mendelian proportions in a mixed population. Science 1908;28(706):49–50.

alleles in a population or identifying disease frequency (q^2). Taking the square root provides q. The equation $1 - q$ gives us p. Once allele frequencies are known, the binomial provides frequencies for homozygous unaffected (p^2), heterozygous carriers (2pq) and those affected (q^2).

The second achievement was (and continues to be) advancing sequencing technology so that the high price tag to sequence the first human genome (0.5–1 billion dollars) decreased precipitously to $1000 or less. With significant funding through the National Human Genome Research Institute (NHGRI), sequencing technology has advanced in such a way that high-throughput sequencing at low cost for an entire exome is now possible.[12,13] All exons (regions of the genome that code amino acids) of a person's genome are collectively called an exome. Sequence data for an entire exome can now be obtained in less than 3 days. The analysis and link to clinical importance (bioinformatics) are now rate-limiting steps that determine clinical utility. Cost, speed, and reproducibility of nucleotide sequence are no longer limiting. Referring to the Rubik cube, in less than 3 decades progress has moved from the green on the axes to the red. These scientific accomplishments moved screening into the multi-dimensional application referred to as ECS.

PURPOSE

The first iteration of panethnic prenatal carrier screening focused on the recessive conditions, cystic fibrosis and spinal muscular atrophy.[14,15] The purpose was to apply genotyping technology to all asymptomatic reproductive-aged women and their partners planning pregnancy or with an early ongoing pregnancy. Screening results can be used to calculate the risk of having a fetus affected by either cystic fibrosis or spinal muscular atrophy. With this information, couples can make reproductive decisions and educate themselves around the needs of children with these disabilities. These two conditions allow risk estimation because they are single-gene recessive disorders with known genetic variants whose allele frequencies are known (**Table 2**). The population carrier frequency (line 1 in **Table 2**) and the detection rate (line 3 in **Table 2**) are the important variables that the determine risk for any recessive condition before screening or after screening.

The latest iteration of panethnic carrier screening incorporates next-generation sequencing (NGS) technology or the ability to sequence across regions of the genome that include genes of interest. The access to more data has changed the focus. Screening now includes not only common recessive conditions but rare recessive conditions, semidominant (eg, factor V Leiden) conditions, and X-linked (eg, fragile X mental retardation) conditions. Importantly, women and their partners may learn they are not only asymptomatic carriers but presymptomatic

Table 2
Example of individual residual and pregnancy risk assessment for cystic fibrosis in northern Europeans

	Description	Formula	Risk
1	Population carrier frequency[a]	—	1/25
2	Pregnancy risk before screening	$1/25 \times 1/25 \times 1/4$	1/2,500
3	Screening DR[b]	—	9/10
4	RR[c]	$1 - DR$	1/10
5	Individual risk after negative screen	$1/25 \times 1/10$	1/250
6	Pregnancy risk after negative screening	$1/250 \times 1/250 \times 1/4$	1/250,000

Abbreviation: DR, detection rate.
    [a] Ethnic specific (eg, northern European, African American, Ashkenazi Jewish).
    [b] Function of number of mutations and population screened, in this case American College of Medical Genetics panel for cystic fibrosis.
    [c] RR is the risk of being a carrier when screening test is negative.

carriers too. For example, young women (<40 years old) identified as carriers of fragile X with 40 to 199 copies of the fragile X mental retardation repeat (CGG) are at risk for premature ovarian failure. This condition was observed in 2.2% to 18.6% of carriers compared with a general population frequency of ~1%. Men with repeats between 55 and 199 are at risk for fragile X–associated ataxia tremor syndrome.[16,17]

Some patients want maximum information (the most genes/conditions and the most variants), whereas others do not. It is critically important that, through counseling, the goals of women and their partners align with the results that will be delivered to them. Some people do not want to know that they are at increased risk for later-onset conditions; they may only want information about fetal risk. Although it is important to know which Rubik cube block most closely meets each person's goals, further refinement may be necessary.

CARRIER FREQUENCY AND RESIDUAL RISK

One benefit patients receive from genetic counseling after screening for single-gene disorders is the calculation of the RR of being a carrier even after receiving negative test results. RR stems from an inability to screen and detect all possible genomic variations in all genes that cause the conditions being screened. Patients who screen negative can have a child affected with the condition being screened because of a failure to recognize or understand variants as pathogenic or decisions not to report all variants. False-negative and false-positive results are a feature of screening tests. Those providing genetic counseling know that all disease-causing variants are not elucidated and convey to patients that results after genetic testing are incomplete. This is true whether low-throughput genotyping or NGS platforms are used.

With the implementation of ECS, RR is difficult to measure and harder for patients and counselors to calculate. The number of conditions screened is large and summation of RR for each condition (*i*) is required. The formula for this summation is: $\sum_{i=1}^{n} RRi$ (where *n* is the number of conditions being screened). Because the frequency of rare population variants is not usually known, the contribution of each to the detection rate (DR) in a general population is not known. RR is a function of the DR (ie, RR=1-DR), the inability to calculate DR and the large number of conditions screened make calculating a meaningful RR elusive (see **Table 2**). In addition, it would be impractical to provide RR estimates for each condition separately during pretest or posttest counseling sessions.

Many companies offer ECS. However, the number of conditions screened and the specific conditions screened for vary. Furthermore, the number of pathogenic variants reported for each condition is not uniform across companies that offer screening; therefore, DR varies across companies. Although laboratories are aware of the criteria used to define variant categories, there are no regulations ensuring that, after NGS, all variants identified and reported are valid. Validating rare variations in the genome can be a difficult task, so the conditions included for reporting and the variants reported are prone to becoming marketing tools and may not always contribute to the goals of population-based carrier screening.

VARIANTS AND CONDITIONS

Variant classification was defined through a joint workshop of the Association of Molecular Pathology and the American College of Medical Genetics and Genomics in 2013.[18] Importantly, the terms mutation (ie, permanent change in the genome) and polymorphism (ie, change in the genome that is present in at least 1% of the population) were eliminated from the current classification system. The term variant replaced both terms and was further divided into a 5-tier classification scheme (**Table 3**). The likely pathogenic and likely benign tiers carry at least 90% certainty.

The driver of conditions that should be reported on carrier screening panels is controversial and ranges from a view that anything that can be reported should be reported to a more conservative view that only conditions that are frequent, severe, and actionable should be included. The problem relates to who defines each of these variables. Without citing data and by consensus, the American Congress of Obstetricians and Gynecologists (ACOG) determined that only conditions with a frequency of 1 in 100 or greater should be included.[19] When health care providers were surveyed, they rated a shortened life span from birth to adolescence and conditions that affect intellectual functioning as the most severe.[20] Actionable conditions are difficult to define. The decisions made by prospective parents once they become aware of an affected pregnancy are personal and range from doing nothing to learning as much as possible before the anticipated birth to pregnancy termination. These actions are likely heterogeneous across regions of the United States. Therefore, until more is learned about the factors that determine how individuals and couples weigh severity and action ability, clinicians are left with a frequency of 1 in 100 (based on no data) as a deterrent to industry marketing strategies.

IMPLEMENTING EXPANDED CARRIER SCREENING

Professional organizations move more slowly compared with the pace of technology. Without advocating for or against ECS, professional organizations coalesced to

Table 3 Nucleotide sequence variation classification	
Pathogenic	Certain
Likely pathogenic	>90% certainty
Uncertain significance	—
Likely benign	>90% certainty
Benign	Certain

provide a framework that can be useful when implementing ECS into clinical practice.[21] There are two basic approaches for prenatal carrier screening:

1. Gene-by-gene screening of a limited number of conditions based on ethnicity
2. ECS, which screens many conditions and variants simultaneously and is panethnic

Advantages and Disadvantages

As the number of conditions and variants reported increases in a screening program, the proportion of people who screen positive also increases. People more often screen positive for something. The advantages of ECS compared with gene-by-gene screening include the opportunity to learn more. Learning more means more information can be shared with family members. Furthermore, identifying presymptomatic risk allows the development of strategies to modify risk and stay informed. For some patients, these are reasons enough to choose ECS. For others, learning more may bring anxiety, especially when presymptomatic conditions are revealed. Anxiety can also emanate from the identification of variants with uncertain significance.

Selection of ECS carries disadvantages beyond potential anxiety. Carrier screening can be performed sequentially (one partner followed by the second based on results) or simultaneously. At baseline, simultaneous screening using NGS costs more than sequential screening. As stated earlier, the probability of at least one member of a couple screening positive is very high when sequential screening is employed, costs increase when a carrier is identified and the partner choses NGS in an effort to learn about all possible variants. This sequence can result in misinformation due to low stringency reporting of variants. Further counseling is often necessary and counseling costs follow laboratory costs. A review of the advantages and disadvantages of gene-by-gene screening compared with ECS is best worked through during pretest counseling.

Counseling

A basic tenet in genetic counseling is to provide nondirective counseling.[22] For this to take place, patients must be educated in a medically literate fashion. All patients should be familiar with the concepts presented in the Rubik cube (see **Fig. 1**), and they should be introduced to the technology platform and that it is imperfect. The concepts of DR and the relationship to RR should be discussed. Effective counseling requires that providers understand the principles of mendelian inheritance. Importantly, the patient's goals when participating in screening should be understood.

ACOG recommends offering panethnic carrier screening for 2 conditions: cystic fibrosis and spinal muscular atrophy. A complete blood count is a general screen for anemia and is a first-line screen for some hemoglobinopathies. Hemoglobin electrophoresis is recommended for patients with African, Mediterranean, Middle Eastern, southeast Asian, or West Indian ancestry. ACOG also recommends offering Ashkenazi Jews screening for Tay-Sachs and Canavan diseases as well as familial dysautonomia.[1]

When patients select screening for more conditions than those recommended by ACOG independent of ethnicity, they are selecting ECS and they may receive results for some conditions that could affect their own health. These conditions include dominant, semidominant, and X-linked conditions. It is not necessary for those who provide pretest counseling to be familiar with the treatment, prognosis, and clinical course of all conditions included on ECS panels.

The hemoglobinopathies represent a group of conditions characterized by abnormalities of alpha or beta chain production or oxygen affinity. The use of molecular testing is associated with a greater RR compared with hemoglobin electrophoresis in screening for hemoglobinopathies, because the pathogenic variants that result in β-thalassemia are often private (specific to families). Furthermore, the genomic changes associated with α-thalassemia are deletions. The most severe α-thalassemia phenotype requires deletions in *cis* (on the same chromosome). Although NGS can determine dosage (the number of copies of a gene), a limitation of NGS is its inability to determine *cis* or *trans* (on opposite chromosomes).

Tay-Sachs disease is often cited as a condition for which NGS is not well suited. Some laboratories use NGS and report the results for 3 common pathogenic variants observed in Ashkenazi Jews. For non–Ashkenazi Jews and in cases in which 1 member of a couple is a known carrier, enzyme analysis is preferred. Because of concerns around ethnic intermixing, enzyme analysis is generally preferred to molecular testing and results in the lowest RR after screening.[21]

There is agreement that the best time to offer carrier screening is before conception. Carrier screening should be offered as early as possible during an ongoing pregnancy. Although sequential screening may be well suited before an ongoing pregnancy, simultaneous screening seems to be the best approach when screening is performed during an established pregnancy.

Importantly, when a family history of a mendelian disorder is identified or already known, referral to a trained genetic professional is indicated. Confirmation of the disorder, genetic variant in the family, and the determination that the familial variant is included on a carrier panel or as part of NGS results is crucial. When the familial variant is not included, special efforts are required to properly inform the concerned couple.

Pretest and Posttest Counseling

NGS used for carrier detection brings uncertainties. A useful approach when providing pretest counseling is to consider the Perceptions of Uncertainties in Genome Sequencing (PUGS) scale framework. Although this scale was introduced as a tool to evaluate patient perceptions of uncertainties in the use of genome sequencing,[23] it highlights the need to address specific areas in pretest and posttest counseling. This scale considers 3 general domains: clinical (ie, health care implications), affective (ie, impact of results on psychosocial health and behavior), and evaluative (whether results are reliable and actionable). These domains translate into important pretest and posttest counseling concerns by patients and reflect areas that should accordingly be discussed (**Tables 4** and **5**).

Table 4		
Pretest counseling using Perceptions of Uncertainties in Genome Sequencing domains		
Domain	**#**	**Consideration by Those Screened**
Clinical	1	Conditions reported have varied severity
Affective	1	Screening is voluntary
	2	Results are confidential and protected by GINA
	3	Plan for returning results
Evaluative	1	Requires accurate paternity information
	2	RR remains after a negative screen
	3	May identify a recessive condition in an asymptomatic person
	4	Asymptomatic carriers of semidominant, dominant, and X-linked disorders may be identified

Abbreviation: GINA, Genetic Information Nondiscrimination Act (signed into US law by President George W. Bush).

Table 5		
Posttest counseling using Perceptions of Uncertainties in Genome Sequencing domains		
Domain	**#**	**Consideration by Those Screened**
Clinical	1	Access to reliable information regarding conditions for which both members of couple screen positive should be provided
Affective	1	A copy of carrier screening results should be provided
	2	Provide written information that can be used for sharing positive screening results with other family members if desired
Evaluative	1	Pregnancies are considered low risk when couples have discordant results (one screens negative and the other positive)
	2	When one partner screens positive and the other negative for Tay-Sachs, the negative partner should be screened with enzyme analysis

SUMMARY

Prenatal carrier screening has expanded to include a larger number of genes and variants offered to all couples with ongoing pregnancy or considering a pregnancy. Panethnic screening for cystic fibrosis and spinal muscular atrophy and screening for a limited number of conditions based on ethnicity are recommended by ACOG. Screening is elective and counseling should be nondirective. As providers offer and patients consider ECS, their goals should align with those of the laboratories used for screening. This process includes consideration of ethnicity, as well genes and variants being reported. Although RR calculations have become an obsolete part of posttest counseling when ECS is selected, it is still important for patients to understand that there is a risk that they may be a carrier for a condition in the setting of a negative screening test result. The PUGS scale offers a useful understanding of the pretest and posttest counseling concerns that should be considered as part of ECS implementation.

REFERENCES

1. ACOG Committee Opinion Summary 691: carrier screening for genetic conditions. Obstet Gynecol 2017;129:597–9.
2. Workshop on Population Screening for the Cystic Fibrosis Gene. Statement from the National Institutes of Health workshop on population screening for the cystic fibrosis gene. N Engl J Med 1990;323:70–1.
3. ACOG Committee Opinion 101: current status of cystic fibrosis carrier screening. Int J Gynaecol Obstet 1992;39:143–5.
4. ACOG Committee Opinion 298: prenatal and preconceptional carrier screening for genetic diseases in individuals of Eastern European Jewish descent. Obstet Gynecol 2004;104:425–8.
5. Lander ES, Linton LM, Birren B, et al. Initial sequencing and analysis of the human genome. Nature 2001;409:860–921.
6. Venter JC, Adams MD, Myers EW, et al. The sequence of the human genome. Science 2001;291:1304–51.
7. Grody WW, Cutting GR, Klinger KW, et al. Laboratory standards and guidelines for population-based cystic fibrosis carrier screening. Genet Med 2001;3:149–54.
8. Watson MS, Cutting GR, Desnick RJ, et al. Cystic fibrosis population carrier screening: 2004 revision of American College of Medical Genetics mutation panel. Genet Med 2004;6:387–91.

9. Abelovich D, Lavon IP, Lerer I, et al. Screening for five mutations detects 97% of cystic fibrosis (CF) chromosomes and predicts a carrier frequency of 1:29 in the Jewish Ashkenazi population. Am J Hum Genet 1992;51:951–6.

10. Kaback MM, Desnick RJ. Hexosaminidase A deficiency. Gene Reviews. 2001. Available at: https://www.ncbi.nlm.nih.gov/books/NBK1218/. Accessed September 30, 2017.

11. Hardy GH. Mendelian proportions in a mixed population. Science 1908;XXVIII: 49–50.

12. Reuter JA, Spacek DV, Snyder MP. High-throughput sequencing technologies. Mol Cell 2015;58:586–97.

13. Heather JM, Chain B. The sequence of sequencers: the history of sequencing DNA. Genomics 2016;107:1–8.

14. American College of Obstetricians and Gynecologists, American College of Medical Genetics. Preconception and prenatal carrier screening for cystic fibrosis; clinical and laboratory guidelines. Washington, DC; Bethesda (MD): ACOG; ACMG; 2001.

15. Prior TW. Carrier screening for spinal muscular atrophy. Genet Med 2008;10: 840–2.

16. Sherman S, Pletcher BA, Driscoll DA. Fragile X syndrome: diagnostic and carrier testing. Genet Med 2005;7(8):584–7.

17. Loesch D, Hagerman R. Unstable mutations in the FMR1 gene and the phenotypes. Adv Exp Med Biol 2012;769:78–114.

18. Richards S, Aziz N, Bale S, et al. Standards and guidelines for the interpretation of sequence variants: a joint consensus recommendation of the American College of Medical Genetics and Genomics and the Association for Molecular Pathology. Genet Med 2015;17(5):405–8.

19. ACOG Committee Opinion Summary 690: carrier screening in the age of genomic medicine. Obstet Gynecol 2017;129:e35–40.

20. Lazarin GA, Hawthorne F, Collins NS, et al. Systematic classification of disease severity for evaluation of expanded carrier screening panels. PLoS One 2014; 9:e114391.

21. Edwards JG, Feldman G, Goldberg J, et al. Expanded carrier screening in reproductive medicine–points to consider: a joint statement of the American College of Medical Genetics and Genomics, American College of Obstetricians and Gynecologists, National Society of Genetic Counselors, Perinatal Quality Foundation, and Society for Maternal-Fetal Medicine. Obstet Gynecol 2015;125:653–62.

22. Rogers CR. Counseling and psychotherapy. Cambridge (MA): Houghton Mifflin; 1942.

23. Biesecker BB, Woolford SW, Klein WMP, et al. PUGS: a novel scale to assess perceptions of uncertainties in genome sequencing. Clin Genet 2017;92:172–9.

Preimplantation Genetic Screening and Preimplantation Genetic Diagnosis

Chantae Sullivan-Pyke, MD, Anuja Dokras, MD, PhD*

KEYWORDS

- Preimplantation genetic screening (PGS) • Preimplantation genetic diagnosis (PGD)
- Comprehensive chromosome screening (CCS) • Next-generation sequencing (NGS)

KEY POINTS

- Preimplantation genetic screening (PGS) improves pregnancy rates by allowing the selection of euploid embryos for transfer. Euploid embryos are more likely to implant and develop into a healthy pregnancy.
- Preimplantation genetic diagnosis (PGD) facilitates the selection of unaffected embryos for transfer to the uterus to avoid transmission of disease-causing genetic mutations.
- Preimplantation embryos can be biopsied at either the cleavage stage or blastocyst stage of development. Blastocyst stage biopsy is advantageous compared with biopsy at the cleavage stage because more cells can be analyzed.
- Currently, comprehensive chromosome screening (CCS) platforms, such as array comparative genomic hybridization (aCGH), single nucleotide polymorphism (SNP) microarray, quantitative polymerase chain reaction (qPCR), and next-generation sequencing (NGS), are used for preimplantation genetic testing (PGT).

INTRODUCTION

Infertility affects 7.5 million women in the United States, and approximately 1 in 8 couples have difficulty conceiving or sustaining a pregnancy.[1] In vitro fertilization (IVF) is a successful treatment of infertility due to several causes, including tubal factor, male factor, and diminished ovarian reserve. Preimplantation genetic testing (PGT) can be performed on cells removed from early embryos before transfer to the uterus (**Fig. 1**)[2] for the purpose of preimplantation genetic diagnosis (PGD) or preimplantation genetic screening (PGS). PGD refers to the detection of known conditions, such as

Disclosure Statement: The authors have no conflicts of interest to disclose.
Division of Reproductive Endocrinology and Infertility, Department of Obstetrics and Gynecology, University of Pennsylvania, 3701 Market Street, Suite 800, Philadelphia, PA 19104, USA
* Corresponding author.
E-mail address: ADokras@obgyn.upenn.edu

Obstet Gynecol Clin N Am 45 (2018) 113–125
https://doi.org/10.1016/j.ogc.2017.10.009
0889-8545/18/© 2017 Elsevier Inc. All rights reserved.

obgyn.theclinics.com

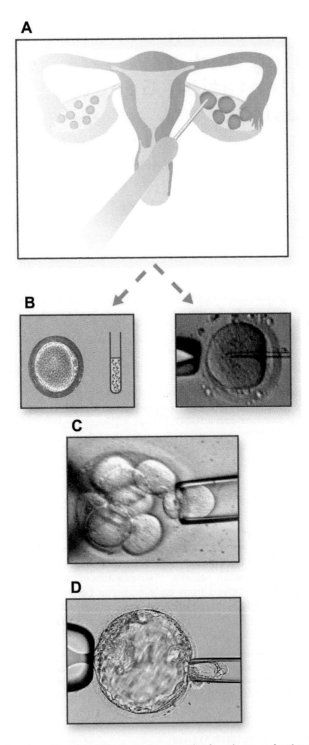

Fig. 1. IVF and embryo biopsy. (*A*) Cartoon showing the female reproductive system. Ovaries are stimulated by daily injections of gonadotropins, and oocytes are then retrieved under

specific mutations or chromosomal rearrangements in embryos, when one or both parents carry a mutation or gene rearrangement. PGS refers to screening for chromosomal aneuploidy, particularly in patients with advanced maternal age or a history of recurrent pregnancy loss. With advances in extended in vitro embryo culture, options for embryo biopsy have advanced from testing of the polar body (PB), 1 to 2 blastomeres at the cleavage stage, to several trophectoderm cells at the blastocyst stage of embryo development. Similarly, there have been significant advances in techniques used for genetic and chromosomal analysis with small amounts of DNA, including polymerase chain reaction (PCR), fluorescence in situ hybridization (FISH), microarray technologies, including single nucleotide polymorphism (SNP) microarrays and array comparative genomic hybridization (aCGH), and next-generation sequencing (NGS).

This article provides an overview of PGT, including advances in embryology and molecular biology, and reviews the advantages and disadvantages of the different techniques in current practice.

BIOPSY TECHNIQUES
Polar Body Biopsy

Polar body (PB) biopsy involves the removal of the first and second PB before embryo cleavage. The clinical use of PB biopsy was first reported in 1990 with no adverse effects on subsequent fertilization rates or development to the cleavage stage.[3] Although PB biopsy avoids the removal of cells from the embryo, it is limited by the fact that only maternal chromosomes or genes can be analyzed, such that the paternal contribution to the embryo cannot be accounted for. In addition, the amount of genetic material obtained from the single cell is small and is subject to limitations, such as allele dropout during PCR. For these reasons, PB biopsy is not widely used.

Cleavage Stage (Blastomere) Biopsy

Embryo biopsy was initially developed at the cleavage stage, in which 1 or 2 blastomeres (cells) are removed from a 6- to 8-cell embryo (see **Fig. 1**C). Blastomere biopsy is advantageous compared with PB biopsy because both maternal and paternal genetic contributions to the embryo can be analyzed. However, the limitations related to the small amount of the genetic material remain, including detection of mosaicism, a potential cause for misdiagnoses.[4] Mosaic rates have been estimated to be as high as approximately 60% at the cleavage stage but are lower, approximately 20%, at the blastocyst stage.[5,6] Furthermore, the removal of cells at the cleavage stage has been shown to slow the development of the embryo to the blastocyst stage and decrease implantation and pregnancy rates.[7–9]

Trophectoderm Biopsy

The first birth after biopsy of trophectoderm cells and blastocyst stage transfer was reported in 2005, a decade after initial reports of births from blastomere biopsy.[10] Development of sequential culture media has allowed for the successful culture of

transvaginal ultrasound guidance. (*B*) Mature oocytes are fertilized with sperm either by combining oocytes and sperm in a dish or by injection of a single sperm into the oocyte directly (intracytoplasmic sperm injection or ICSI). (*C*) Embryos may be biopsied on day 3 of embryo culture (cleavage stage). A single cell is removed from the embryo with a biopsy pipette and sent for PGT. (*D*) Embryos may also be biopsied on day 5 of embryo culture (blastocyst stage). A few trophectoderm cells are biopsied and sent for PGT. ([*C, D*] *From* IVFMD. Fertility treatments. Available at: http://ivfmd.net/fertility-treatments/pgs/. Accessed October 18, 2017; with permission.)

embryos to the blastocyst stage and improved pregnancy rates after blastocyst transfer.[11,12] Subsequently, trophectoderm biopsy was applied in clinical practice, allowing multiple cells to be biopsied (see **Fig. 1**D) and subsequent improvements in the accuracy of the results with decreased amplification errors.[13,14] Excellent concordance between inner cell mass and the trophectoderm has been shown using SNP array for analysis.[15] Although a lower rate of mosaicism has been described at the blastocyst stage compared with the cleavage, confined mosaicism within this layer as described in the placenta at later stages or variations within the trophectoderm itself can lead to erroneous results.[16] Few IVF centers with in-house laboratories may be able to perform blastocyst biopsy, genetic analysis, and transfer during the same IVF cycle.[17] However, in most centers the biopsied cells are sent to a reference laboratory for analysis, which necessitates cryopreservation of the blastocyst after biopsy and transfer of unaffected embryos in a subsequent cycle.

PREIMPLANTATION GENETIC SCREENING

Since the first IVF birth in 1978, different technologies, such as intracytoplasmic sperm injection (ICSI), extended culture to the blastocyst stage and cryopreservation have been developed to improve pregnancy rates. However, the high proportion of aneuploidy noted in human embryos results in decreased implantation rates or early pregnancy losses. It is estimated that up to 50% of pregnancy losses in the first trimester are due to embryonic aneuploidy.[18] Aneuploidy increases with maternal age and is an important consideration as women delay childbearing and are typically older when they seek fertility treatments.[19] Pregnancy rates can therefore be improved by transferring only euploid embryos into the uterus, resulting in a higher implantation rate and lower miscarriage rate. PGS is an option for any patient undergoing IVF, but is particularly useful for couples in whom the female partner is of advanced reproductive age, those with a medical history of recurrent first-trimester pregnancy losses, and those with recurrent implantation failure in prior IVF cycles.

PREIMPLANTATION GENETIC SCREENING PLATFORMS

Fluorescent in situ hybridization (FISH) was initially used with blastomere biopsy to evaluate a limited number of chromosomes most frequently associated with aneuploidy.[20,21] However, development of single-cell whole genome amplification has allowed the use of newer technologies that can quantify all 24 chromosomes, also known as comprehensive chromosome screening (CCS). CCS technologies include microarray technology with single nucleotide polymorphism (SNP) arrays, comparative genome hybridization (aCGH) arrays, quantitative polymerase chain reaction (qPCR), and next-generation sequencing (NGS) (**Table 1**).

Array Comparative Genomic Hybridization Microarray

Conventional comparative genome hybridization (CGH) was the first of the CCS methods to become widely available and involved isolation and fluorescent labeling of DNA obtained from a blastomere biopsy and compared with DNA from a karyotypically normal individual. Both test and reference DNA were then hybridized to a normal metaphase chromosome spread for about 3 to 5 days.[22] Conventional CGH was replaced by microarray-based CGH (aCGH), which involves hybridizing DNA to a microarray[23] with approximately 3000 to 4000 human DNA fragments, and the intensity of both hybridization signals relative to each probe is measured as log2Ratio.[21,23] aCGH has a resolution up to 10 Mb,[24] allowing detection of whole chromosome aneuploidy and segmental aneuploidies larger than 10 Mb. A limitation of aCGH is the

Table 1
Comparison of complete chromosome screening methods

Methods	Cost of Initial Investment	Complexity	Duration (h)	Abnormalities Detected	Limitations	Resolution
aCGH	Medium	Medium	~12	Whole chromosome aneuploidy Translocations	False positives Unable to detect mosaicism	Medium
SNP microarray	High	High	Up to 72	Whole chromosome aneuploidy Parental origin Translocations	Inability to detect balanced chromosomal rearrangements Inability to detect mosaicism	High
qPCR	Low	Low	4	Whole chromosome aneuploidy	Not designed to detect segmental aneuploidy Unable to detect mosaicism or translocations	Low
NGS	High	High	<24	Whole chromosome aneuploidy Mosaicism, mitochondrial copy number Single-gene disorders Translocations	Limited ability to detect balanced chromosome translocations	High

universal cutoff used to assign aneuploidy status to all chromosomes instead of chromosome-specific cutoffs, which may lead to false positives.[25] In addition, aCGH was developed to investigate cancer genetics with larger quantities of DNA that hybridize to the array for about 72 hours, compared with the small quantities available for PGS and shorter hybridization time, ~4 to 12 hours. The small quantity of DNA available for PGS could also contribute to the error rate for aCGH for PGS estimated at about 2% to 5%.[25,26] Trophectoderm biopsy with aCGH has been shown to be highly sensitive (98.8%) and specific (99.6%) for chromosomal aneuploidy screening.[25]

Single Nucleotide Polymorphism Microarray

Single nucleotide polymorphism (SNP) microarrays detect pairs of single nucleotides in genomic DNA that are highly variable within a given species. An array typically evaluates approximately 300,000 SNPs spaced throughout the genome[27] and provides a genotype for each sample compared with a reference genome, thereby identifying whole chromosome aneuploidy, approximately 250 common structural aberrations, and uniparental disomy.[21,23] SNP arrays can also be used for molecular cytogenetics to detect the ratio of intensity of the B-to-A alleles at heterozygous loci, allowing the detection of deletions and duplications with high resolution.[23] Some of the limitations of SNP microarrays include limited ability to detect structural abnormalities less than 5 Mb, an inability to detect balanced chromosome rearrangements, and genetic abnormalities in a consanguineous couple may not be detected because SNPs may be homozygous at every locus.[21,28–30] Furthermore, SNP arrays for PGS have been found to be time consuming, costly, and complex.

Quantitative Polymerase Chain Reaction

Quantitative polymerase chain reaction (qPCR) was developed as a more rapid method to identify 24-chromosome aneuploidy and has been validated for analysis of trophectoderm biopsies.[17,23] In this method, there is a preamplification step, followed by multiplex PCR on the sample directly to amplify at least 2 sequences on each arm of each chromosome.

The advantages of qPCR include short analysis time of approximately 4 hours, allowing for embryo transfer in the same IVF cycle. Chromosome-specific cutoffs are used for each chromosome, thereby resulting in high diagnostic accuracy of 98.6%.[17,25] The error rate after CCS by qPCR has been shown to be as low as 0.21% per embryo designated as euploid.[31] Limitations of qPCR-based aneuploidy screening include the fact that it has not been validated with blastomere and PB biopsy samples. qPCR is also limited by the small number of samples that can be run simultaneously.[17,23] qPCR is also unable to detect segmental aneuploidy.[17]

Next-Generation Sequencing

Next-generation sequencing (NGS) for PGS includes whole genome amplification of DNA followed by library preparation with tagging and fragmentation of the input DNA before PCR.[32] There are currently 2 major platforms for NGS, Illumina MiSeq (Illumina Inc., San Diego, CA) and Thermo Fisher Ion PGM (Thermo Fisher Scientific, Waltham, MA).[33,34] Both platforms are benchtop sequencers with fast turnover and targeted clinical applications but use different sequencing techniques.[35]

Illumina MiSeq is based on sequencing by synthesis, in which single bases are detected by a fluorescent label as they are incorporated into the growing DNA strands. MiSeq can identify whole chromosome aneuploidy, mosaicism, and mitochondrial copy number and may also allow for screening for single-gene disorders and translocations.[21,36] Segmental imbalances of ~14 Mb and greater can be detected,[32,36] and the overall error rate has been reported to be 0.8%.[37] Thermo Fisher Ion PGM uses semiconductor sequencing technology in which a proton is released when a nucleotide is incorporated into the growing DNA strand. The proton release triggers a change in pH that is detected by an ion-sensitive field-effect transistor sensor, which transmits electrical pulses to a computer that translates them into a DNA sequence.[38] Unbound nucleotides are then washed off before a different base is added. PGM does not require fluorescence or camera scanning, thereby decreasing cost and size of the machine and facilitating fast sequencing.[35] PGM can identify whole chromosome aneuploidy, deletions or duplications to a resolution of approximately 800 kb to 1 Mb, mosaicism, mitochondrial copy number, and single-gene disorders[21,39] with an overall error rate of 1.71%.[37] The sensitivity and specificity of NGS for the detection of aneuploid chromosome number are 100% and 99.98%, respectively.[36]

The use of NGS was clinically validated in a double-blind prospective PGS trial comparing NGS with aCGH after trophectoderm biopsy.[32] Paired comparison between the 2 techniques revealed 99.5% concordance (95% confidence interval [CI] 96.8–99.9).[32] Excellent clinical pregnancy rates and ongoing implantation rates of 63.8% and 62.0%, respectively, were also noted with the transfer of euploid blastocysts after testing by both aCGH and NGS.[32] Compared with aCGH, NGS also has the potential advantages of reduced cost caused by high-throughput sequencing and the ability to sequence many samples simultaneously, increased automation, improved detection of partial or segmental aneuploidies, and the detection of mosaicism.[32]

The ability of NGS to detect mosaicism was demonstrated in a case-control study in which amplified DNA samples from blastocysts identified as euploid by aCGH, and resulting in either miscarriage or live birth, were reanalyzed by NGS.[18] Of the blastocysts diagnosed as euploid by aCGH that resulted in miscarriage, 13.6% were diagnosed as mosaic and 5.2% were diagnosed as polyploid by NGS.[18] It is also important to note that some embryos diagnosed as mosaic have resulted in successful live births.[18,40] Given that embryos diagnosed as mosaic by NGS are more likely to end in miscarriage than successful pregnancies, the transfer of mosaic embryos requires additional counseling.[41] Although NGS is a powerful platform for CCS, there are limitations, including an inability to detect balanced chromosome translocations and difficulties with interpretation of segmental aneuploidies secondary to artifacts related to whole genome amplification.[32]

PREGNANCY RATES AFTER PREIMPLANTATION GENETIC SCREENING

To clinically validate the technologies used in PGS, it is crucial to evaluate ongoing pregnancy and live birth rates. Relative to untested blastocysts, the transfer of euploid blastocysts confirmed by aCGH after day 3 biopsy has shown improved implantation rates (52.8% vs 27.6%) and live birth rates per transfer (64.7% vs 27.4%).[42] When compared with single-embryo transfer without CCS, in a retrospective study, the use of trophectoderm biopsy with rapid qPCR and subsequent single embryo transfer resulted in higher ongoing pregnancy rates (55.0% vs 41.8%) and lower miscarriage rates (10.5% vs 24.8%).[43] In a randomized controlled trial with 72 patients who underwent CCS with qPCR, implantation rates were higher in the CCS group (79.8%) compared with controls (63.2%) (relative risk [RR] 1.26; 95% CI 1.04–1.39; $P = .002$), and the percent with a live birth was 66.4% and 47.9%, respectively (RR 1.39; 95% CI 1.07–1.60; $P = .001$).[44] Furthermore, in a study involving 88,010 singleton live births after IVF cycles with PGD (n = 439) or without PGD (n = 87,571), there was no increased risk of adverse perinatal outcomes in PGD cycles.[45] There is also no demonstrable impact of blastomere biopsy on growth parameters, birth weight, hospitalizations, or congenital malformations in children followed to 2 years of age.[46,47] These studies demonstrate the safety and efficacy of PGT in IVF cycles as well as excellent pregnancy outcomes after testing.

PREIMPLANTATION GENETIC DIAGNOSIS
Early Indications

Preimplantation Genetic Diagnosis (PGD) is used to detect specific mutations or chromosomal rearrangements in embryos before uterine transfer. Gardner and Edwards[48] first reported in 1968 the feasibility of accurately predicting the sex of rabbits after biopsy of trophectoderm cells at the blastocyst stage. This initial animal study set the stage for later studies involving the biopsy and PGD of human embryos. The first successful case of PGD in humans was performed in 1990 for adrenoleukodystrophy, an X-linked recessive condition. Embryos were biopsied at the cleavage stage, and PCR was performed to detect a repetitive sequence on the Y chromosome to distinguish male and female embryos. Female embryos were selected for transfer resulting in 2 ongoing pregnancies.[20] In 1992, PGD was first applied to detect a specific mutation associated with cystic fibrosis (F508), an autosomal recessive disease, after biopsy of cleavage stage embryos resulting in a live birth.[49]

Other indications for PGD include carriers of Robertsonian and reciprocal translocations who are at a higher risk of infertility and miscarriage. Reciprocal translocations are the most common structural abnormality for which PGD is offered.[50] PGD also facilitates the option of nondisclosure in adult onset conditions, such as Huntington disease, which is the ability to test embryos without parents having to know their own carrier status. Other conditions that may be diagnosed by PGD are listed in **Box 1**.

Single Gene Disorders and Karyomapping

Conventional methods for PGD relied on PCR-based technologies to amplify DNA segments and identify specific mutation or linked polymorphisms for single-gene disorders, including autosomal dominant and recessive conditions, sex-linked dominant and recessive, and FISH for translocations. This process is time consuming because it requires the development of probes to detect specific candidate markers within the family and could take 3 to 4 months.[30] SNP-based technology and NGS have become the preferred methods today.

Karyomapping uses genome-wide linkage analysis to compare SNPs in the couple to those from family members of known genetic status to identify the combination of SNP alleles associated with a chromosome carrying the gene mutation.[51] Karyomapping, therefore, significantly reduces the time to develop a patient-specific test. After whole genome amplification and genotyping, karyomaps are constructed, and informative parental SNPs are identified. The genotypes of the embryos are compared with a reference genome (typically that of an affected family member), and the parental origin of the affected or unaffected genes is determined.[52] Karyomapping has been shown to be highly accurate with 97.7% concordance with conventional PGD without the need to design patient- or disease-specific tests.[30] Although karyomapping is expensive compared with PCR-based technology, the cost is balanced by the decreased workup time and skilled labor costs.[30]

ETHICAL CONSIDERATIONS

As discussed, all existing methods of PGS and diagnosis have an error rate, and the risk of transferring abnormal embryos must be balanced against the risk of discarding normal embryos. In addition, the implications of a mosaic result after PGT of the trophectoderm layer are unclear with few reports of live births after the transfer of mosaic

Box 1
Genetic diseases that may be diagnosed by preimplantation genetic diagnosis

Autosomal dominant conditions

Familial adenomatous polyposis

Huntington disease

BRCA1/BRCA2 mutations

Retinoblastoma

Kell antigen

Myotomic dystrophy

Peutz-Jeghers syndrome

Limb girdle muscular dystrophy

Hereditary multiple osteochondromas

Dilated cardiomyopathy

Lynch syndrome

Crouzon disease

Polycystic kidney disease

Brugada syndrome

Multiple endocrine neoplasia

Autosomal recessive conditions

Sickle cell disease

Spinal muscular atrophy

Joubert syndrome

Ornithine transcarbamylase deficiency

Osteogenesis imperfecta

Gaucher disease

Fanconi anemia

Propionic acidemia

Alpha-1 antitrypsin deficiency

Cystic fibrosis

Homocystinuria

Usher syndrome

Familial dysautonomia

Methylmalonic acidemia

X-linked

Duchenne muscular dystrophy

Becker muscular dystrophy

Chronic granulomatous disease

Fragile X syndrome

X-linked adrenoleukodystrophy

embryos.[40] Although PGT was developed to prevent genetic disease in offspring and improve pregnancy rates, it has the potential of being abused to discriminate and select against disability.[53] Providers must discuss all options with patients before proceeding with IVF and PGT to ensure they are well-counseled.

SUMMARY

Preimplantation genetic testing (PGT) has revolutionized IVF and the treatment of infertility, because it enables the transfer of euploid embryos that are unaffected by deleterious mutations or chromosomal rearrangements that parents may carry. Euploid embryos are more likely to implant and result in a successful pregnancy compared with aneuploid or mosaic embryos; therefore, the ability to detect embryo ploidy status has led to improved pregnancy rates. Several platforms are available for comprehensive chromosome screening (CCS) but vary in terms of their complexity, cost, and time investment. Platforms based on next-generation sequencing (NGS) are becoming standard of care because of high accuracy and high throughput. Patients should also be counseled that PGT methods have an inherent error rate and do not replace routine prenatal screening. Embryo transfer should proceed with embryos diagnosed as euploid before the transfer of any mosaic embryo because of unclear counseling guidelines regarding mosaicism. Segmental chromosomal aneuploidy detected by NGS may be real or artifactual; therefore, caution must be exercised in the interpretation of this result. Testing should therefore take place in conjunction with a genetic counselor. With continued research, preimplantation genetic screening (PGS) and preimplantation genetic diagnosis (PGD) applications will further expand with high accuracy and financial accessibility to patients.

REFERENCES

1. Sunderam S, Kissin DM, Crawford SB, et al. Assisted reproductive technology surveillance–United States, 2013. MMWR Surveill Summ 2015;64(11):1–25.
2. Practice Committee of Society for Assisted Reproductive Technology, Practice Committee of American Society for Reproductive Medicine. Preimplantation genetic testing: a Practice Committee opinion. Fertil Steril 2008;90(5): S136–43.
3. Verlinsky Y, Ginsberg N, Lifchez A, et al. Analysis of the first polar body: preconception genetic diagnosis. Hum Reprod 1990;5(7):826–9.
4. Treff NR, Franasiak JM. Detection of segmental aneuploidy and mosaicism in the human preimplantation embryo: technical considerations and limitations. Fertil Steril 2017;107(1):27–31.
5. Capalbo A, Wright G, Elliott T, et al. FISH reanalysis of inner cell mass and trophectoderm samples of previously array-CGH screened blastocysts shows high accuracy of diagnosis and no major diagnostic impact of mosaicism at the blastocyst stage. Hum Reprod 2013;28(8):2298–307.
6. Johnson DS, Gemelos G, Baner J, et al. Preclinical validation of a microarray method for full molecular karyotyping of blastomeres in a 24-h protocol. Hum Reprod 2010;25(4):1066–75.
7. De Vos A, Staessen C, De Rycke M, et al. Impact of cleavage-stage embryo biopsy in view of PGD on human blastocyst implantation: a prospective cohort of single embryo transfers. Hum Reprod 2009;24(12):2988–96.
8. Mastenbroek S, Twisk M, van Echten-Arends J, et al. In vitro fertilization with preimplantation genetic screening. N Engl J Med 2007;357(1):9–17.

9. Scott RT Jr, Upham KM, Forman EJ, et al. Cleavage-stage biopsy significantly impairs human embryonic implantation potential while blastocyst biopsy does not: a randomized and paired clinical trial. Fertil Steril 2013;100(3):624–30.

10. Kokkali G, Vrettou C, Traeger-Synodinos J, et al. Birth of a healthy infant following trophectoderm biopsy from blastocysts for PGD of β-thalassaemia major: case report. Hum Reprod 2005;20(7):1855–9.

11. Gardner DK, Vella P, Lane M, et al. Culture and transfer of human blastocysts increases implantation rates and reduces the need for multiple embryo transfers. Fertil Steril 1998;69(1):84–8.

12. Jones GM, Trounson AO, Gardner DK, et al. Evolution of a culture protocol for successful blastocyst development and pregnancy. Hum Reprod 1998;13(1): 169–77.

13. Dokras A, Sargent IL, Ross C, et al. Trophectoderm biopsy in human blastocysts. Hum Reprod 1990;5(7):821–5.

14. Veiga A, Sandalinas M, Benkhalifa M, et al. Laser blastocyst biopsy for preimplantation diagnosis in the human. Zygote 1997;5(4):351–4.

15. Johnson DS, Cinnioglu C, Ross R, et al. Comprehensive analysis of karyotypic mosaicism between trophectoderm and inner cell mass. Mol Hum Reprod 2010;16(12):944–9.

16. Gleicher N, Vidali A, Braverman J, et al. Accuracy of preimplantation genetic screening (PGS) is compromised by degree of mosaicism of human embryos. Reprod Biol Endocrinol 2016;14(1):54.

17. Treff NR, Tao X, Ferry KM, et al. Development and validation of an accurate quantitative real-time polymerase chain reaction–based assay for human blastocyst comprehensive chromosomal aneuploidy screening. Fertil Steril 2012;97(4): 819–24.

18. Maxwell SM, Colls P, Hodes-Wertz B, et al. Why do euploid embryos miscarry? A case-control study comparing the rate of aneuploidy within presumed euploid embryos that resulted in miscarriage or live birth using next-generation sequencing. Fertil Steril 2016;106(6):1414–9.e5.

19. Franasiak JM, Forman EJ, Hong KH, et al. The nature of aneuploidy with increasing age of the female partner: a review of 15,169 consecutive trophectoderm biopsies evaluated with comprehensive chromosomal screening. Fertil Steril 2014;101(3):656–63.e1.

20. Handyside AH, Kontogianni EH, Hardy K, et al. Pregnancies from biopsied human preimplantation embryos sexed by Y-specific DNA amplification. Nature 1990;344(6268):768–70.

21. Brezina PR, Anchan R, Kearns WG. Preimplantation genetic testing for aneuploidy: what technology should you use and what are the differences? J Assist Reprod Genet 2016;33(7):823–32.

22. Wilton L, Williamson R, McBain J, et al. Birth of a healthy infant after preimplantation confirmation of euploidy by comparative genomic hybridization. N Engl J Med 2001;345(21):1537–41.

23. Handyside AH. 24-Chromosome copy number analysis: a comparison of available technologies. Fertil Steril 2013;100(3):595–602.

24. Illumina. 24sure Microarray Pack. Product information sheet. April 14, 2014. Available at: https://www.illumina.com/content/dam/illumina-marketing/documents/products/product_information_sheets/product-info-24sure.pdf. Accessed July 2, 2017.

25. Capalbo A, Treff NR, Cimadomo D, et al. Comparison of array comparative genomic hybridization and quantitative real-time PCR-based aneuploidy screening of blastocyst biopsies. Eur J Hum Genet 2015;23(7):901–6.

26. Rodrigo L, Mateu E, Mercader A, et al. New tools for embryo selection: comprehensive chromosome screening by array comparative genomic hybridization. Biomed Res Int 2014;2014:517125.

27. Illumina. HumanCytoSNP-12 v2.1 BeadChip data sheet. March 22, 2016. Available at: https://www.illumina.com/content/dam/illumina-marketing/documents/products/datasheets/cytosnp-12-data-sheet-1570-2016-003.pdf. Accessed June 22, 2017.

28. Rauch A, Ruschendorf F, Huang J, et al. Molecular karyotyping using an SNP array for genomewide genotyping. J Med Genet 2004;41(12):916–22.

29. Slater HR, Bailey DK, Ren H, et al. High-resolution identification of chromosomal abnormalities using oligonucleotide arrays containing 116,204 SNPs. Am J Hum Genet 2005;77(5):709–26.

30. Natesan SA, Bladon AJ, Coskun S, et al. Genome-wide karyomapping accurately identifies the inheritance of single-gene defects in human preimplantation embryos in vitro. Genet Med 2014;16(11):838–45.

31. Werner MD, Leondires MP, Schoolcraft WB, et al. Clinically recognizable error rate after the transfer of comprehensive chromosomal screened euploid embryos is low. Fertil Steril 2014;102(6):1613–8.

32. Fiorentino F, Bono S, Biricik A, et al. Application of next-generation sequencing technology for comprehensive aneuploidy screening of blastocysts in clinical preimplantation genetic screening cycles. Hum Reprod 2014;29(12):2802–13.

33. MiSeqTM. System specification sheet: sequencing. May 17, 2016. Available at: https://www.illumina.com/content/dam/illumina-marketing/documents/products/datasheets/datasheet_miseq.pdf. Accessed June 22, 2017.

34. System ion personal genome machine™ (PGM™) System. Available at: https://www.thermofisher.com/order/catalog/product/4462921. Accessed June 22, 2017.

35. Liu L, Li Y, Li S, et al. Comparison of next-generation sequencing systems. J Biomed Biotechnol 2012;2012:251364.

36. Fiorentino F, Biricik A, Bono S, et al. Development and validation of a next-generation sequencing-based protocol for 24-chromosome aneuploidy screening of embryos. Fertil Steril 2014;101(5):1375–82.

37. Quail MA, Smith M, Coupland P, et al. A tale of three next generation sequencing platforms: comparison of Ion Torrent, Pacific Biosciences and Illumina MiSeq sequencers. BMC Genomics 2012;13:341.

38. Pennisi E. Semiconductors inspire new sequencing technologies. Science 2010;327(5970):1190.

39. Treff NR, Fedick A, Tao X, et al. Evaluation of targeted next-generation sequencing–based preimplantation genetic diagnosis of monogenic disease. Fertil Steril 2013;99(5):1377–84.e6.

40. Greco E, Minasi MG, Fiorentino F. Healthy babies after intrauterine transfer of mosaic aneuploid blastocysts. N Engl J Med 2015;373(21):2089–90.

41. PGDIS position statement on chromosome mosaicism and preimplantation aneuploidy testing at the blastocyst stage. July 19, 2016. Available at: http://www.pgdis.org/docs/newsletter_071816.html. Accessed April 5, 2017.

42. Rubio C, Bellver J, Rodrigo L, et al. In vitro fertilization with preimplantation genetic diagnosis for aneuploidies in advanced maternal age: a randomized, controlled study. Fertil Steril 2017;107(5):1122–9.

43. Forman EJ, Tao X, Ferry KM, et al. Single embryo transfer with comprehensive chromosome screening results in improved ongoing pregnancy rates and decreased miscarriage rates. Hum Reprod 2012;27(4):1217–22.
44. Scott RT Jr, Upham KM, Forman EJ, et al. Blastocyst biopsy with comprehensive chromosome screening and fresh embryo transfer significantly increases in vitro fertilization implantation and delivery rates: a randomized controlled trial. Fertil Steril 2013;100(3):697–703.
45. Sunkara SK, Antonisamy B, Selliah HY, et al. Pre-term birth and low birth weight following preimplantation genetic diagnosis: analysis of 88 010 singleton live births following PGD and IVF cycles. Hum Reprod 2017;32(2):432–8.
46. Desmyttere S, De Schepper J, Nekkebroeck J, et al. Two-year auxological and medical outcome of singletons born after embryo biopsy applied in preimplantation genetic diagnosis or preimplantation genetic screening. Hum Reprod 2009; 24(2):470–6.
47. Desmyttere S, De Rycke M, Staessen C, et al. Neonatal follow-up of 995 consecutively born children after embryo biopsy for PGD. Hum Reprod 2012;27(1): 288–93.
48. Gardner RL, Edwards RG. Control of the sex ratio at full term in the rabbit by transferring sexed blastocysts. Nature 1968;218(5139):346–9.
49. Handyside AH, Lesko JG, Tarin JJ, et al. Birth of a normal girl after in vitro fertilization and preimplantation diagnostic testing for cystic fibrosis. N Engl J Med 1992;327(13):905–9.
50. De Rycke M, Belva F, Goossens V, et al. ESHRE PGD consortium data collection XIII: cycles from January to December 2010 with pregnancy follow-up to October 2011. Hum Reprod 2015;30(8):1763–89.
51. Gimenez C, Sarasa J, Arjona C, et al. Karyomapping allows preimplantation genetic diagnosis of a de-novo deletion undetectable using conventional PGD technology. Reprod Biomed Online 2015;31(6):770–5.
52. Handyside AH, Harton GL, Mariani B, et al. Karyomapping: a universal method for genome wide analysis of genetic disease based on mapping crossovers between parental haplotypes. J Med Genet 2010;47(10):651–8.
53. Ouellette A. Selection against disability: abortion, ART, and access. J Law Med Ethics 2015;43(2):211–23.

Key Ethical Issues in Prenatal Genetics
An Overview

Ruth M. Farrell, MD, MA[a],*, Megan A. Allyse, PhD[b]

KEYWORDS

- Ethical issues • Clinical translation • Genetic tests • Informed consent
- Patient decision making

KEY POINTS

- The clinical integration of new prenatal genetic technologies raises important medical and ethical considerations for patients, families, healthcare providers and systems, and society.
- It is critical that effective strategies are put in place to ensure that patients and families make informed decisions about the use of new prenatal genetic tests.
- Despite advances in genetics and obstetrics, inherent challenges to the use of reproductive genetic technologies in utero persist.

INTRODUCTION

The clinical integration of prenatal genetic technologies raises important medical and ethical considerations for patients, families, health care providers, health care systems, and society. Prenatal genetic technologies can have a significant positive impact on health care decisions, health care quality, safety, and access. At the same time, these tests are associated with important ethical issues, such as informed consent, information disclosure, and actionability, and larger societal implications regarding illness and disability. This article outlines some of the lead issues associated with prenatal genetic screens and diagnostic tests. The goal of this overview is not to produce a comprehensive inventory of the ethical issues associated with prenatal genetic testing but to touch on some of the major points to consider when integrating new genetic science and technology into prenatal care.

Disclosure Statement: Neither author has any conflict of interest to disclose.
[a] OB/GYN and Women's Health Institute, Department of Bioethics, Cleveland Clinic, 9500 Euclid Avenue, A-81, Cleveland, OH 44195, USA; [b] Center for Bioethics, Mayo Clinic, 200 1st Street Southwest, Rochester, MN 55905, USA
* Corresponding author.
E-mail address: farrelr@ccf.org

Obstet Gynecol Clin N Am 45 (2018) 127–141
https://doi.org/10.1016/j.ogc.2017.10.006
0889-8545/18/© 2017 Elsevier Inc. All rights reserved.

CHALLENGES INHERENT WITH GENETIC TESTING IN UTERO

The advent of genetic technologies has made possible new medical achievements in the diagnosis and treatment of disease. Although there are promising efforts under way to achieve personalized genomic medicine, there are important ethical questions that must be addressed if such efforts are to maximize benefits to patients.[1–4] Any such challenges are amplified in the context of prenatal care. In this setting, the information gained from genetic tests may lead to critical health care decisions that can affect the course and outcome of the pregnancy; the decision-making process entails not only understanding the current implications but also forecasting notions of health, well-being, and quality of life months and years in the future and doing so with respect to values and beliefs.[5–8] For some women, this may entail the decision to end a pregnancy if a serious genetic condition is identified. For others, this information might be used with the intention to continue the pregnancy and prepare for the birth of a child with a serious medical condition.[9,10] In addition, such information can influence future reproductive decisions, including deciding if, when, or how to achieve another pregnancy using assisted reproductive technologies (eg, preimplantation genetic diagnosis [PGD] and/or donor gametes) or whether other family-building efforts take precedence (eg, adoption and/or foster care).[11] Thus, it is critical for resources to be in place that allow pregnant patients to engage with prenatal genetic technologies in a way that is informed and meets their needs, goals, and values, both now and as the technology evolves, as a way that makes it possible to gain an unpredicted volume of genetic information about the pregnancy.[12,13] Yet, there are many challenges associated with achieving this benchmark, raising concerns about the ethical implications that arise when women use or decline such tests in absence of meaningful pretest and post-test decision making.[14]

One of the challenges that must be considered pertains to the difficulty of correlating genotype with phenotype. Because of the nature of pregnancy and the fact that key clinical information cannot be obtained until after birth, there is an inherent lack of prognostic uncertainty that comes with the use of genetic tests in the prenatal care context. In the case of newborn or adult testing, information gained from genetic testing is combined with an individual's phenotypic information to help determine a prognosis. Yet, in the context of prenatal medicine, genetic tests must be interpreted with only limited phenotypic information.[12,15] Although advances in fetal imaging do provide a better picture of fetal anatomy, including more precise approaches to ultrasound and the use of other imaging modalities, such as MRI, critical clinical information related to outcome and prognosis is frequently required to understand test results in the context of the newborn's morphology.

Another challenge is the scientific and technical limitations associated with genetic testing itself, specifically limitations in the ability to interpret test results. Tests using next-generation sequencing technology can provide detailed information about genomic variants; however, although some identifiable variants are well characterized, others may be associated with a variant of uncertain significance or a rare genetic condition in which the disease progression in not well known.[15–17] Even with the newest advances, such as cell-free DNA (cfDNA) technology, there is still the potential for uncertainty in the process of assessing fetal risk as a woman may receive a false-positive, false-negative, or inconclusive result. This can cause a chain of difficult and potentially troubling decisions women who undergo utilize this new screen.[18–20] Limitations may also be encountered in settings where genetic testing is performed to investigate a finding of multiple fetal anomalies. In such cases, the approach to genetic testing may be based on a health care provider's suspicion of the different possible syndromes that could cause these anomalies. The selected panel, however, may not include the causative chromosome or locus for study, often leading to more questions than answers. Thus, important questions may remain unanswered while new ones are raised in the testing process, leading to uncertainty about how best to optimize pregnancy outcomes.

Even in the context of a known genetic condition, variable penetrance and expressivity, coupled with biological and environmental factors, can affect the severity and course of a disease over an individual's lifetime, although these may be mitigated by specialized medical care and services, such as physical therapy and occupational therapy. It is also important to recognize that there are changes taking place in communities and social infrastructures to provide greater support for individuals with physical and cognitive disabilities. All these factors can add to uncertainty in the interpretation of the severity of a genetic variant identified in utero.

Challenges to informed decision making not only a function of technological factors but also are inherent in the information needs of the pregnant woman, which include the values, preferences, and needs of both her and her family.[8,21,22] For some women, prenatal screening tests remain a preferable way to obtain information about the pregnancy because they are devoid of the procedural complications or risks associated with chorionic villus sampling or amniocentesis. Until recently, these screening modalities were limited to serum analyte screens and anatomic ultrasound, each of which has a known false-positive and false-negative rate that requires diagnostic confirmation. The advent of cfDNA has had a significant impact on the delivery of prenatal care because it can screen for a larger number of chromosomal and subchromosomal variants with increased accuracy.[20,23] Yet, despite advances in cfDNA technology, there continues to be ongoing need to interpret individualized risk based on the incidence of that condition in the general population.[23–25] Based on women's values and needs, however, some prefer to receive only risk information through noninvasive screening tests and decline additional diagnostic procedures to investigate an abnormal screen result.[26] Thus, for the foreseeable future, there will be persistent uncertainty characterizing women's decision making that must be acknowledged and addressed in the informed decision-making and consent process.

TECHNOLOGICAL CONSIDERATIONS: IN THEORY AND IN REALITY

The growing capability of prenatal molecular diagnostics opens the door to prenatally discover several genetic conditions beyond the traditional aneuploidies, including those historically offered in the setting of adult testing (eg, predictive and presymptomatic testing) but increasingly emerging in the reproductive context (eg, PGD for BRCA testing).[27] This raises important ethical questions about which conditions should be included on testing panels and the implications of those choices for women, families, communities, and society.[28,29] At the same time, it raises important ethical questions about concepts of health and illness, ability and disability, and the role of health care and health care providers in the construction of those concepts. The question of which genetic traits should be the focus of prenatal testing has been repeatedly raised, notably by the disability community, who voice concerns about the impact of such decisions on individuals and communities. Disability advocates have argued that the mere act of looking for a certain genetic trait during the prenatal period suggests it as a viable, and perhaps desirable, target for decisions about pregnancy termination.[30] The Down syndrome community has been among the most vocal in this regard.[31] In particular, the community has pushed back against the universal offer of prenatal screening for Down syndrome as an implication that society would be better without individuals with Down syndrome.[31-34] A leading concern is that the decision to include tests for this chromosomal aneuploidy and facilitate prenatal testing for the condition sends a clear message to individuals and families living with Down syndrome that their existence is undesirable.[35-37] These debates have set the stage for further debate as prenatal genetic testing expands to identify other genetic variants. As diagnostic testing shifts from karyotype to microarray to whole-exome sequencing and as cfDNA screening moves in a similar direction, more genetic conditions become candidates for these decisions and conversations about the limits, if any, of prenatal information become more complicated.

Actionability

One of the most commonly discussed issues relates to actionability and what actions may be taken in light of prenatal genetic information.[38,39] This may include specific actions, ranging from the decision to end a pregnancy to the pursuit of medical interventions to mitigate the downstream effects of a genetic condition. This may also include broader notions of preparation of the self, home, and family for the birth of a child with a serious medical condition. In some conditions, in particular those involving structural abnormalities, such as myelomeningocele, prenatal interventions, such as fetal surgery, have shown some benefit in limiting the severity of postnatal symptoms for the child. In addition, the prenatal identification of affected newborns can influence plans for the timing, location, and mode of delivery. There remains, however, debate about how actionability can be complicated and problematized in situations of when patients have limited access to tertiary care centers to manage high-risk pregnancies and deliveries. In cases of experimental procedures medical insurance may decline to cover intensive interventions, leaving them beyond the reach of some families.

Severity

Another criterion that has been suggested for evaluating the genetic conditions that should be prioritized in the prenatal setting is the projected severity of the phenotype.[40] The primary question raised pertains to who defines severity and how this concept is defined. Although there is variation in how this concept is construed, one definition addresses outcomes for a child with respect to compatibility with life or with a life independent of significant medical interventions.[41] Tay-Sachs disease, for instance, has generally been considered a severe condition because it is lethal in young children and, in the process of disease progression, commonly involves considerable pain and suffering for the child. Other conditions, however, seem to raise more debate. In high-resource settings, individuals with what were previously thought to be serious and life-limiting conditions, including sickle cell disease, cystic fibrosis, and Down syndrome, may now live well into adulthood, although not without significant access to medical care. Furthermore, some families who live with what might be considered a disabling condition — whether congenital or acquired — report high quality of life[42,43] This may lead many patient, healthcare providers, and communities to question whether these conditions should be designated as serious. This emphasize the need for adequate counseling and decision-making mechanisms to assist patients in conceptualizing this concept within their own family.[44]

The other aspect of severity that is difficult to define is penetrance. Conditions with widely variable penetrance can be difficult to define as either severe or not severe because severity is entirely dependent on phenotype expression. For example, aneuploidies of the sex chromosomes, including Turner syndrome and Klinefelter syndrome, have widely variable penetrance. Although some individuals with these conditions have sufficiently mild phenotypes that they may remain undiagnosed for decades or only diagnosed when difficulties with fertility occur; others may have more involved medical, cognitive, or behavioral sequelae Although these conditions are included in many cfDNA screening panels, there is considerable debate about the justification for their inclusion in such panels.

Age of Onset

A third criterion that is often discussed is the age at which symptoms of a genetic condition are likely to occur. Many researchers and scholars in the field argue that conditions, including Huntington disease, Parkinson disease, or BRCA-related breast cancer, should be critically appraised before being included in prenatal testing panels. Although they are often life limiting, late-onset conditions theoretically allow individuals to live full lives for the first several decades. Three dominant arguments can be made to question the appropriateness of screening for late-onset conditions.[45] One argument is that terminating a pregnancy that would otherwise develop into an individual with a (presumably) healthy and productive life span of several decades is not warrented, given all that an individual might experience and contribute during that time. Another argument is that, if the goal of screening for these conditions is to allow individuals to be prepared or empower them to make health care decisions, it would be more appropriate to provide screening (if desired) in early adulthood.[46] Finally, there may be treatments in the future to arrest the development of disease or mitigate its symptoms.[47] Nevertheless, families of individuals with severe late-onset conditions frequently report that such conditions can be devastating to both an individual and to family members and, thus, have a vested interest in avoiding that outcome.[48,49] Thus, there is a position that late-onset conditions may be appropriate for preventative genetic screening, such as PGD or preconception carrier screening, but less so for prenatal genetic screening, such as cfDNA screening or reporting on prenatal microarray.[50–52]

Parental Autonomy

An additional consideration with respect to genetic conditions included on testing panels is that there are no externally applied criteria that can or should define the acceptability or lack of acceptability in screening or testing for a genetic condition. To do so would be to assume a universal definition of quality of life and circumstances that is both impractical and undesirable.[53] In much the same way that any individual termination decision is intensely contextual and personalized, so too should the decision about the fetal information that may be accessed and the subsequent prenatal choices based on that information. A condition that may not be considered serious by a family may be different when considered by a family that already has one or more children affected by a genetic condition[54] or limited financial or medical-social resources to provide adequate care for a child with a severe or complicated heath problem. This view suggests that genetic information about the fetus should be stripped of the normative weighting inherent in defining something as severe and instead allow parents to weight the Information independently. This would also distance health care providers, policy makers, and test manufacturers from the task of determining which conditions should or should not be included; all information that is technically feasible would be made available to parents, who would select the information that is relevant or desirable to their decision making.[55]

Practical solutions to how this could be accomplished are a subject of debate.[56] Some commentators have suggested that there should be a menu of conditions among which prospective parents could select, although how those panels would be constructed (ie, all serious conditions, lethal conditions, and all actionable conditions) returns to questions of what the medical and social definitions of those terms should be.[41] Another possibility is to take an all-or-nothing approach, in which a pregnant woman and partner could decide whether any prenatal genetic information would be likely to change prenatal decisions and, if not, opt out of receiving any genetic screening or testing prenatally. Although this is, effectively, the approach that has historically applied to prenatal screening, it presents two main issues. The first pertains to routinization of screening. This approach describes the gradual acceptance of screening tests as a component of standards of prenatal care delivery, either in the form of a serum screen (eg, maternal serum analytes or cfDNA screening) or anatomic ultrasound.[57] The concern is that, in this context, patients have to take concerted efforts in declining such screens once offered and, as a result, may undergo screening or testing despite their values and preferences against receiving that information.[58] The second issue pertains to prediction and an individual's ability to individualize implications over time. For instance, when individuals are asked how a disability would affect their quality of life, they routinely report that it would have a negative impact. When individuals who have been disabled are questioned, however, they regularly report a high quality of life. Thus, it is difficult for prospective parents to know how much personal utility prenatal genetic information might have before they receive it. Research also reports that individual beliefs about the permissibility of pregnancy termination do not significantly map to choices if a fetal abnormality is identified. Thus, it is not clear how prospective parents would be prepared to exercise their autonomy.

Access and Regulatory Factors

The utility of any of these approaches is proscribed by the social and regulatory environment in which they are introduced. Some systems, such as the Human Fertilisation and Embryology Authority, allow for centralized control of the applications of prenatal genetics based on a combination of normative determinations about the acceptability of certain technology applications and resource allocation of scarce health care resources in a closed, single-payer health system. In general, however, prenatal genetic technologies have developed largely outside existing regulatory controls. The US Food and Drug Administration has chosen for decades not to regulate laboratory developed tests, which include carrier screens, cfDNA screens, prenatal microarray panels, and applications of PGD. The result is that, in the United States and many other areas of the world, the content of prenatal genetic panels is determined by technical feasibility and market demand.[59] In the past, a relatively stable arrangement between public health systems, academic research, and industry actors resulted in the gradual translation of emerging clinical research into clinical practice through a system of industry-funded and academically implemented clinical trials. The involvement of public health systems allowed for some normative input into the necessary or desirable scope of screening and required technologies to demonstrate both clinical effectiveness and cost effectiveness to justify their implementation.

New prenatal genetic technologies, by contrast, have largely circumvented this system and operate almost exclusively under competitive private-sector models.[59] Individual laboratories or medical practices are relatively free to decide which genetic screens they are or are not willing to conduct, and market forces routinely encourage widening the scope of that testing. One of the most controversial examples is the use of PGD to identify fetal sex. Although some parents argue that this is desirable for family-balancing purposes, the practice is widely controversial due to its possible use by individuals from cultural backgrounds that may prioritize one sex over another. In the United States, however, the practice is not proscribed and private clinics do offer it. Another area of expansion has been developments in optimal donor matching in third-party reproduction. Companies now offer services in which prospective parent DNA is matched to find gamete donors that are most likely to result in a child with the desired profile. There are no restrictions, however, that constrain such services to matching based on the possibility of severe conditions only. Thus, it may be that in many areas, the parental autonomy model is the only likely response to the question of what should and should not be an appropriate target of prenatal genetic information.

CLINICAL CONSIDERATIONS: INFORMED DECISION MAKING AND CONSENT

Given the challenges inherent in the clinical application of prenatal genetic technologies, it is critical that robust structures are in place to ensure that patients can make informed, value-centered decisions about their options, including whether to undergo testing, what scope of information to acquire, and the possible range of actions to take based on that information.[8,60] This process is important not only for the course and outcome of the current pregnancy but also for future reproductive decision making; information gained from prenatal screening and testing may affect decisions about whether to initiate future pregnancies and how to approach family-building efforts (eg, in vitro fertilization with PGD, donor gametes, and adoption). It is also critical for the health and well-being of the pregnant woman, a function not only of the psychological and emotional consequences but also of the medical sequelae of interventions taken in response to genetic information (eg, termination or antenatal procedures). Finally, such information may also have an impact on the rest of the family, specifically, on living children who may learn of a genetic condition in the process.

Informed decision making and informed consent are the cornerstones of this process. These are process by which patients acquire information about their screening and testing options and make informed, value-driven choices about whether to accept or decline.[61,62] The best way to facilitate informed decision making for prenatal screening and testing, however, particularly as the content of panel tests increases, has long been a subject of debate. And, although critically important, there remain important gaps in knowledge of how to achieve these processes in the obstetric setting, where decisions may be heavily laden with complexity, uncertainty, and considerations of values.[63]

Advances in prenatal genetic tests pose specific challenges to this process. First, there is the issue of patient knowledge and information delivery. There is ongoing debate about the nature and level of detail of information that should be disclosed to patients.[54] This is superimposed on preexisting barriers to women accessing the information and support needed to make informed choices about their testing options.[64–67] There is also the issue of timing and whether all or only a portion of information about relevant testing options should be delivered in the pretest or post-test context. Because information about risk is central to such discussions, there are also questions about how to best communicate concepts of risk and uncertainty to patients, concepts that are traditionally among the most difficult to communicate and conceptualize in informed-consent discussions.[68] These include information pertinent not only to the pregnancy but also to the health of the pregnant woman because cfDNA screening may also reveal malignancy or other health issues within the woman.[7] In addition, these processes must address accurate concepts of risk, a notion grounded in preexisting paradigm that designated women as low-risk or high-risk for a fetal genetic condition based primarily on maternal age, an approach that had greater applicability before prenatal tests included microdeletions and other genomic variants that are not associated with advanced maternal age.[69,70]

Second, there is the issue of who should present and discuss this information with patients. Because of the complex and value-based nature of information gained from genetic testing, it is strongly preferable to have a specialist in prenatal genetics provide pretest and post-test counseling. Ideally, this includes a certified genetic counselor and/or maternal-fetal medicine specialist with specific training in the conduct and clinical interpretation of genetic information. Due to the limited number of available specialists, however, counseling is more frequently falling to primary obstetricians.[70–72] Furthermore, although most obstetricians are familiar with serum screening regimes for prenatal screening, they may have less experience in counseling with more complicated testing panels or less time in the clinical visit to do so. Some commercial laboratories have addressed this shortage by using genetic counselors who offer to counsel patients about a company's proprietary testing platform.[73] Although this is an approach that may bridge health care personnel shortages in the clinical sector, there are potential biases and conflicts of interest that could arise in this setting.

Finally, there is an issue of autonomous, voluntary decision making and informed consent with the integration of new genetic technologies.[57,74–76] The increasing routinization of prenatal genetic testing into prenatal care delivery has raised concerns about women's ability to decline testing if such fetal health information is not desired or valued.[77–79] Additionally, as it becomes increasingly possible to acquire a large volume of genetic information from analysis of maternal serum (currently cfDNA and anticipated whole fetal cell analysis), there is growing concern that pregnant women will face unprecedented health care and social pressures to accept testing.[80–82] Thus, the informed decision and consent process should contain mechanisms for women to decline or defer decisions about undergoing prenatal screening and testing.

ACCESS TO CARE

Disparities in access to pregnancy care, and resulting disparities in maternal/fetal outcomes, have long been documented; in the United States, such disparities are strongly correlated with maternal race and ethnicity and socioeconomic status.[83–85] This trend has been linked to differential outcomes among mothers and children among certain populations, especially low socioeconomic status groups.[86,87] Although these existing issues raise salient ethical issues of justice broadly, there are specific considerations related to access to prenatal genetic tests.

One issue pertains to financial barriers to prenatal testing services. Although US states have made concerted efforts to support universal access to traditional screening mechanisms — such as combined or sequential screening —these services vary considerably by state. Only one state, California, is currently known to include cfDNA screening in its public health screening program, and then only as a contingent screen after high-risk first-trimester screening. Similarly, state Medicaid programs have taken widely variable approaches to coverage of cfDNA screening. For many Medicaid programs, diagnostic testing is already a covered service and can be made available with fewer out-of-pocket costs for patients than newer cfDNA screens, a factor that also affects patient decision making about which tests are available and acceptable to them.[88,89] Even among individuals who have access to private insurance, coverage of cfDNA screens is inconsistent. Due to the competitive nature of the genetic testing market,[88] many private insurance companies and commercial testing providers make proprietary pricing arrangements with specific providers that can have a drastic impact on out-of-pocket cost of a cfDNA screen,[90] depending on the indications and the brand name of the test in question. Lacking insurance coverage, many patients cannot afford the out-of-pocket cost of cfDNA screening, which can range into the thousands of dollars.[91]

These trends are exacerbated by recent efforts by some interest groups to remove pregnancy care from the list of conditions health insurance providers are required to cover. If patients are forced to make hard choices between higher premiums to cover prenatal care and other financial priorities, the number of women who have access to robust prenatal care is likely to decline. Inevitably, disparate access leads to a tiered system in which some pregnant women are making more informed decisions about pregnancy management and subsequent care than others.

Another key issue pertains to the location and number of prenatal genetic specialists who have the knowledge and clinical infrastructure to support patient counseling and provide testing services.[92] Many women, in particular those in rural or other limited-resource areas, may have access primarily to primary obstetric clinics or other community-based health organizations in which prenatal screening is not available or, if it is available, may have no or limited specialized educational and counseling support.[93] Thus, individuals in traditionally underserved urban and rural communities face more pervasive barriers to receive comprehensive counseling about their prenatal screening and testing options. When available, in many areas, access to specialty follow-up care, including genetic counseling or consultation with a maternal fetal medicine specialist, is subject to delay in diagnosis and prenatal care planning.[94]

Although not all patients use prenatal genetic tests with the notion of terminating a pregnancy identified with a genetic condition, abortion is a critical part of the picture in discussions about prenatal genetic testing.[92] Thus, it is necessary to consider the rapidly declining access to termination services in many parts of the United States. In the past few years, there have been several changes that have either defunded or led to the closing of many prenatal care providers, including abortion providers.[93] In some states, there are no longer any practitioners who provide abortion services and only 1 or 2 providers in the country provide later-term abortion services.[94] This affects all women but particularly women who already face barriers to early prenatal care access and experience delay in diagnosis of a fetal genetic anomaly until the second trimester with subsequent ramifications for accessing abortion services when sought.[94] Women seeking termination of an affected pregnancy are frequently faced with the high cost of traveling to access services, with the accompanying implications not only for ongoing employment, impact on existing family, and finances but also for health risks associated with later-term abortions, notably those performed by undertrained or understaffed health care facilities, which may be the only accessible resources for some patients. Ethical issues related to abortion are an international issue. There is also the issue of offering prenatal screening and diagnostic testing in other parts of the world where abortion is legally banned or culturally shunned for the entire community, even in situations where families lack sufficient medical and psychosocial resources do not exist to support the care of a child with a serious medical condition, unless individuals and families have the means to travel to access them.[95]

SUMMARY

The development and clinical translation of new prenatal genetic technologies raise important ethical issues for patients, providers, families, and society. Some of the lead ethical issues have remained constant and unresolved since the early days of pre- natal genetic screening and diagnostic testing, although now amplified in the setting of advances in genetic science and technology. Other ethical issues are either just emerging or becoming better defined with the growing capability to identify details within the fetal genome. Given the nature and pace of prenatal technology, it is critical that ethical considerations go hand in hand with the medical aspects of testing to ensure that such technologies can benefit the women, families, and communities who elect for their use.

REFERENCES

1. Bush LW, Rothenberg KH. Dialogues, dilemmas, and disclosures: genomic research and incidental findings. Genet Med 2012;14:293–5.
2. Juengst E. Genetic testing and the moral dynamics of family life. Public Underst Sci 1999;8:1–13.
3. Clayton EW. Ethical, legal, and social implications of genomic medicine. N Engl J Med 2003;349:562–9.
4. Khoury MJ, Gwinn M, Yoon PW, et al. The continuum of translation research in genomic medicine: how can we accelerate the appropriate integration of human genome discoveries into health care and disease prevention? Genet Med 2007;9: 665–74.
5. Minear MA, Alessi S, Allyse M, et al. Noninvasive prenatal genetic testing: current and emerging ethical, legal, and social issues. Annu Rev Genomics Hum Genet 2015;16:369–98.
6. Lyerly AD, Mitchell LM, Armstrong EM, et al. Risks, values, and decision making surrounding pregnancy. Obstet Gynecol 2007;109:979–84.
7. Kuppermann M, Nease RF, Learman LA, et al. Procedure-related miscarriages and Down syndrome-affected births: implications for prenatal testing based on women's preferences. Obstet Gynecol 2000;96:511–6.
8. American College of Obstetricians and Gynecologists, Society for Maternal-Fetal Medicine. Practice bulletin no. 163 summary: screening for fetal aneuploidy. Ob- stet Gynecol 2016;127:979–81.
9. Mattheis PJ, Hickey F, Tinkle BT, et al. Prenatal diagnosis: beyond decisions about termination. J Pediatr 2008;153:728.
10. Ralston SJ, Wertz D, Chelmow SD, et al. Pregnancy outcomes after prenatal diag- nosis of aneuploidy. Obstet Gynecol 2001;97:729–33.
11. Downing C. Negotiating responsibility: case studies of reproductive decision- making and prenatal genetic testing in families facing Huntington disease. J Genet Couns 2005;14:219–34.
12. Bianchi DW. From prenatal genomic diagnosis to fetal personalized medicine: progress and challenges. Nat Med 2012;18:1041–51.
13. Bianchi DW, Platt LD, Goldberg JD, et al. Genome-wide fetal aneuploidy detec- tion by maternal plasma DNA sequencing. Obstet Gynecol 2012;119:890–901.
14. Committee on Ethics, American College of Obstetricians and Gynecologists, Committee on Genetics, American College of Obstetricians and Gynecologists. ACOG committee opinion no. 410: ethical issues in genetic testing. Obstet Gyne- col 2008;111:1495–502.

15. Wapner RJ, Driscoll DA, Simpson JL. Integration of microarray technology into prenatal diagnosis: counselling issues generated during the NICHD clinical trial. Prenat Diagn 2012;32:396–400.
16. Bernhardt BA, Soucier D, Hanson K, et al. Women's experiences receiving abnormal prenatal chromosomal microarray testing results. Genet Med 2013; 15:139–45.
17. Marteau TM, Kidd J, Michie S, et al. Anxiety, knowledge and satisfaction in women receiving false positive results on routine prenatal screening: a random-ized con-trolled trial. J Psychosom Obstet Gynaecol 1993;14:185–96.
18. Walser SA, Werner-Lin A, Russell A, et al. "Something extra on chromosome 5": parents' understanding of positive prenatal chromosomal microarray analysis (CMA) results. J Genet Couns 2016;25:1116–26.
19. American College of Obstetricians and Gynecologist Committee on Genetics. Committee opinion no. 545.Noninvasive prenatal testing for fetal aneuploidy. Obstet Gynecol 2012;120:1532–4.
20. Gregg AR, Skotko BG, Benkendorf JL, et al. Noninvasive prenatal screening for fetal aneuploidy, 2016 update: a position statement of the American College of Medical Genetics and Genomics. Genet Med 2016;18:1056–65.
21. Allyse M, Sayres LC, Goodspeed T, et al. "Don't want no risk and don't want no problems": public understandings of the risks and benefits of non-invasive prena-tal testing in the United States. AJOB Empir Bioeth 2015;6:5–20.
22. Farrell RM, Agatisa PK, Nutter B. What women want: lead considerations for cur-rent and future applications of noninvasive prenatal testing in prenatal care. Birth 2014;41:276–82.
23. American College of Obstetricians and Gynecologist Committee on Genetics and the Society for Maternal-Fetal Medicine. Committee opinion no. 640: cell-free DNA screening for fetal aneuploidy. Obstet Gynecol 2015;126:e31–7.
24. Bianchi DW, Simpson JL, Jackson LG, et al. Fetal gender and aneuploidy detec-tion using fetal cells in maternal blood: analysis of NIFTY data. National Institute of Child Health and Development Fetal Cell Isolation study. Prenat Diagn 2002;22: 609–15.
25. Mennuti MT, Cherry AM, Morrissette JJ, et al. Is it time to sound an alarm about false-positive cell-free DNA testing for fetal aneuploidy? Am J Obstet Gynecol 2013;209:415–9.
26. Werner-Lin A, Barg FK, Kellom KS, et al. Couple's narratives of communion and isolation following abnormal prenatal microarray testing results. Qual Health Res 2016;26:1975–87.
27. Wright C, Hall A, Burton H, et al. Cell-free fetal nucleic acids for non-invasive pre-natal diagnosis. Report of the UK expert working group. London: PHG Founda-tion; 2009.
28. Deans Z, Clarke AJ, Newson AJ. For your interest? The ethical acceptability of using non-invasive prenatal testing to test 'purely for information'. Bioethics 2015;29:19–25.
29. Kaposy C. Noninvasive prenatal whole-genome sequencing: a solution in search of a problem. Am J Bioeth 2017;17:42–4.
30. Parens E, Asch A. The disability rights critique of prenatal genetic testing. Reflec-tions and recommendations. Hastings Cent Rep 1999;29:S1–22.
31. Alderson P. Prenatal screening, ethics and Down's syndrome: a literature review. Nurs Ethics 2001;8:360–74.
32. Asch A, Wasserman D. Reproductive testing for disability. The Routledge com-panion to bioethics. New York: Taylor and Francis; 2014. p. 417.

33. Saxton M. Why members of the disability community oppose prenatal diagnosis and selective abortion. In: Parens, Asch, editors. Prenatal testing and disability rights. Washington, DC: Georgetown University Press; 2000. p. 147–64.

34. van Schendel RV, Kater-Kuipers A, van Vliet-Lachotzki EH, et al. What do parents of children with Down syndrome think about non-invasive prenatal testing (NIPT)? J Genet Couns 2017;26:522–31.

35. Parens E, Asch A. Disability rights critique of prenatal genetic testing: reflections and recommendations. Ment Retard Dev Disabil Res Rev 2003;9:40–7.

36. Wasserman D, Asch A. The uncertain rationale for prenatal disability screening. Virtual Mentor 2006;8:53–6.

37. Cole R, Jones G. Testing times: do new prenatal tests signal the end of Down syndrome? N Z Med J 2013;126:96–102.

38. Conley Ii WK, McAdams DC, Donovan GK, et al. Beneficence in utero: a framework for restricted prenatal whole-genome sequencing to respect and enhance the well-being of children. Am J Bioeth 2017;17:28–9.

39. Botkin JR, Francis LP, Rose NC. Concerns about justification for fetal genome sequencing. Am J Bioeth 2017;17:23–5.

40. Strong C. Tomorrow's prenatal genetic testing: should we test for 'minor' diseases? Arch Fam Med 1993;2:1187–93.

41. Wilfond BS. Breaking the sounds of silence: respecting people with disabilities and reproductive decision making. Am J Bioeth 2017;17:37–9.

42. Skotko BG, Levine SP, Macklin EA, et al. Family perspectives about Down syndrome. Am J Med Genet A 2016;170A:930–41.

43. Skotko BG, Levine SP, Goldstein R. Having a son or daughter with Down syndrome: perspectives from mothers and fathers. Am J Med Genet A 2011;155A:2335–47.

44. Farrell RM, Nutter B, Agatisa PK. Meeting patients' education and decision-making needs for first trimester prenatal aneuploidy screening. Prenat Diagn 2011;31(13):1222–8.

45. de Jong A, Dondorp WJ, Frints SG, et al. Advances in prenatal screening: the ethical dimension. Nat Rev Genet 2011;12:657–63.

46. Ensenauer RE, Michels VV, Reinke SS. Genetic testing: practical, ethical, and counseling considerations. Mayo Clin Proc 2005;80:63–73.

47. Erez A, Plunkett K, Sutton VR, et al. The right to ignore genetic status of late onset genetic disease in the genomic era; prenatal testing for Huntington disease as a paradigm. Am J Med Genet A 2010;152A:1774–80.

48. Kastrinos F, Stoffel EM, Balmaña J, et al. Attitudes toward prenatal genetic testing in patients with familial adenomatous polyposis. Am J Gastroenterol 2007;102:1284–93.

49. Milner KK, Han T, Petty EM. Support for the availability of prenatal testing for neurological and psychiatric conditions in the psychiatric community. Genet Test 1999;3:279–86.

50. Evers-Kiebooms G, Harper P, Zoeteweij MW. Prenatal testing for late-onset neurogenetic diseases. Oxford (United Kingdom): BIOS Scientific Publishers; 2003.

51. Offit K, Sagi M, Hurley K. Preimplantation genetic diagnosis for cancer syndromes: a new challenge for preventive medicine. JAMA 2006;296:2727–30.

52. Wang C-W, Hui EC. Ethical, legal and social implications of prenatal and preimplantation genetic testing for cancer susceptibility. Reprod Biomed Online 2009;19:23–33.

53. Munthe C. A new ethical landscape of prenatal testing: individualizing choice to serve autonomy and promote public health: a radical proposal. Bioethics 2015; 29:36–45.
54. Wertz DC, Rosenfield JM, Janes SR, et al. Attitudes toward abortion among parents of children with cystic fibrosis. Am J Public Health 1991;81:992–6.
55. Chen SC, Wasserman DT. A framework for unrestricted prenatal whole-genome sequencing: respecting and enhancing the autonomy of prospective parents. Am J Bioeth 2017;17:3–18.
56. Allyse M, Evans JP, Michie M. Dr. Pangloss's clinic: prenatal whole genome sequencing and a return to reality. Am J Bioeth 2017;17:21–3.
57. Suter SM. The routinization of prenatal testing. Am J Law Med 2002;28:233–70.
58. Seavilleklein V. Challenging the rhetoric of choice in prenatal screening. Bioethics 2009;23:68–77.
59. Agarwal A, Sayres LC, Cho MK, et al. Commercial landscape of noninvasive prenatal testing in the United States. Prenat Diagn 2013;33:521–31.
60. Farrell RM, Agatisa PK, Mercer MB, et al. Balancing risks: the core of women's deci- sions about noninvasive prenatal testing. AJOB Empir Bioeth 2015;6:42–53.
61. Berg J, Appelbaum P. Informed consent: legal theory and clinical practice. New York: Ox-ford University Press; 2001.
62. Faden RR, Beauchamp TL. A history of informed consent. New York: Oxford University Press; 1986.
63. Edmonds BT. Shared decision-making and decision support: their role in obstetrics and gynecology. Curr Opin Obstet Gynecol 2014;26:523–30.
64. van den Berg M, Timmermans DR, ten Kate LP, et al. Informed decision making in the context of prenatal screening. Patient Educ Couns 2006;63:110–7.
65. Marteau TM, Dormandy E. Facilitating informed choice in prenatal testing: how well are we doing? Am J Med Genet 2001;106:185–90.
66. Farrell RM, Agatisa PK, Mercer MB, et al. The use of noninvasive prenatal testing in obstetric care: educational resources, practice patterns, and barriers reported by a national sample of clinicians. Prenat Diagn 2016;36(6):499–506.
67. Bianchi DW, Chudova D, Sehnert AJ, et al. Noninvasive prenatal testing and incidental detection of occult maternal malignancies. JAMA 2015;314:162–9.
68. Pauker SP, Pauker SG. Prenatal diagnosis–Why is 35 a magic number? N Engl J Med 1994;330:1151–2.
69. Cleary-Goldman J, Morgan MA, Malone FD, et al. Screening for Down syndrome: practice patterns and knowledge of obstetricians and gynecologists. Obstet Gynecol 2006;107:11–7.
70. Farrell RM, Agatisa PK, Nutter B. Patient-centered prenatal counseling: aligning obstetric healthcare professionals with needs of pregnant women. Women Health 2015;55:280–96.
71. Sayres LC, Allyse M, Norton ME, et al. Cell-free fetal DNA testing: a pilot study of obstetric healthcare provider attitudes toward clinical implementation. Prenat Diagn 2011;31:1070–6.
72. Stoll KA, Mackison A, Allyse MA, et al. Conflicts of interest in genetic counseling: acknowledging and accepting. Genet Med 2017. https://doi.org/10.1038/gim. 2016.216.
73. van den Heuvel A, Chitty L, Dormandy E, et al. Will the introduction of noninvasive prenatal diagnostic testing erode informed choices? An experimental study of health care professionals. Patient Educ Couns 2010;78:24–8.
74. Press N, Browner CH. Why women say yes to prenatal diagnosis. Soc Sci Med 1997;45:979–89.

75. Charo RA, Rothenberg KH. The good mother. In: Apple R, Golden J, Rothenberg KH, et al, editors. Women and prenatal testing: facing the challenges of genetic technology. Columbus (OH): Ohio State University Press; 1994. p. 105–13.

76. Deans Z, Newson AJ. Should non-invasiveness change informed consent procedures for prenatal diagnosis? Health Care Anal 2011;19:122–32.

77. Marteau TM, Slack J, Kidd J, et al. Presenting a routine screening test in antenatal care: practice observed. Public Health 1992;106:131–41.

78. Lippman A. The genetic construction of prenatal testing: choice, consent, or conformity for women?. In: Apple R, Golden J, Rothenberg KH, et al, editors. Women and prenatal testing: facing the challenges of genetic technology. Columbus (OH): Ohio State University Press; 1994. p. 9–34.

79. Johnston J, Farrell RM, Parens E. Supporting women's autonomy in next-generation prenatal testing. JAMA 2017;377(6):505–7.

80. Schmitz D, Netzer C, Henn W. An offer you can't refuse? Ethical implications of non-invasive prenatal diagnosis. Nat Rev Genet 2009;10:515.

81. Dickens BM. Ethical and legal aspects of noninvasive prenatal genetic diagnosis. Int J Gynaecol Obstet 2014;124:181–4.

82. Suther S, Kiros GE. Barriers to the use of genetic testing: a study of racial and ethnic disparities. Genet Med 2009;11:655–62.

83. Bryant AS, Worjoloh A, Caughey AB, et al. Racial/ethnic disparities in obstetric outcomes and care: prevalence and determinants. Am J Obstet Gynecol 2010; 202:335–43.

84. Markens S. 'I'm not sure if they speak to everyone about this option': analyzing disparate access to and use of genetic health services in the US from the perspective of genetic counselors. Crit Publ Health 2016;16:1–14.

85. Phillippi JC. Women's perceptions of access to prenatal care in the United States: a literature review. J Midwifery Womens Health 2009;54:219–25.

86. Lu MC, Kotelchuck M, Hogan VK, et al. Innovative strategies to reduce disparities in the quality of prenatal care in under-resourced settings. Med Care Res Rev 2010;67(5 Suppl):198S–230S.

87. Pergament D, Ilijic K. The legal past, present and future of prenatal genetic testing: professional liability and other legal challenges affecting patient access to services. J Clin Med 2014;3:1437–65.

88. de Jong A, de Wert GM. Prenatal screening: an ethical agenda for the near future. Bioethics 2015;29:46–55.

89. Mozersky J, Mennuti MT. Cell-free fetal DNA testing: who is driving implementation? Genet Med 2013;15:433–4.

90. Prince AE. Prevention for those who can pay: insurance reimbursement of genetic-based preventive interventions in the liminal state between health and disease. J Law Biosci 2015;2:365–95.

91. Mikat-Stevens NA, Larson IA, Tarini BA. Primary-care providers' perceived barriers to integration of genetics services: a systematic review of the literature. Genet Med 2015;17:169–76.

92. Ballantyne A, Newson A, Luna F, et al. Prenatal diagnosis and abortion for congenital abnormalities: is it ethical to provide one without the other? Am J Bioeth 2009;9:48–56.

93. Jones RK, Zolna MR, Henshaw SK, et al. Abortion in the United States: incidence and access to services, 2005. Perspect Sex Reprod Health 2008;40:6–16.

94. Farrell RM, Mabel H, Reider MW, et al. Implications of Ohio's 20-week abortion ban on prenatal patients and the assessment of fetal anomalies. Obstet Gynecol 2017;129:795–9.
95. Bernabé-Ortiz A, White PJ, Carcamo CP, et al. Clandestine induced abortion: prevalence, incidence and risk factors among women in a Latin American country. CMAJ 2009;180:298–304.

The Status of Genetic Screening in Recurrent Pregnancy Loss

 CrossMark

Daniel Kaser, MD

KEYWORDS

- Aneuploidy • Comprehensive chromosomal screening • Inversion • Miscarriage
- Products of conception • IVF • Preimplantation genetic screening
- Spontaneous abortion

KEY POINTS

- Recurrent pregnancy loss (RPL) is often idiopathic. Approximately 50% of cases have a discernible cause.
- Numerical chromosomal abnormalities in the conceptus are primarily due to maternal meiotic nondisjunction, and the rate and complexity of embryonic aneuploidy are primarily driven by female age.
- Structural chromosomal abnormalities (balanced translocations or inversions) can lead to unbalanced gametes depending on specific recombination and segregation patterns during meiosis. The attendant reproductive risk depends on the type of rearrangement and its parental origin.
- Products of conception may be analyzed by cytogenetics, array comparative genomic hybridization, or single nucleotide polymorphism microarray. Each platform has its respective advantages and disadvantages.
- Preimplantation genetic screening decreases the likelihood of subsequent miscarriage per euploid embryo transfer, but further investigation is required to define the time to viable pregnancy, cumulative live birth rates, and cost of treatment as compared with expectant management.

INTRODUCTION

Spontaneous abortion or miscarriage is defined as the loss of pregnancy before 20 weeks' gestation. Although miscarriage is common, occurring in 15% to 25% of all clinically recognized pregnancies, recurrent pregnancy loss (RPL), defined as the loss of 2 or more clinical pregnancies, is uncommon. It is estimated that approximately

Conflicts of Interest: None.
Funding Source: None.
Reproductive Medicine Associates of New Jersey, 140 Allen Road, Basking Ridge, NJ 07920, USA
E-mail address: dkaser@rmanj.com

Obstet Gynecol Clin N Am 45 (2018) 143–154
https://doi.org/10.1016/j.ogc.2017.10.007
0889-8545/18/© 2017 Elsevier Inc. All rights reserved.

obgyn.theclinics.com

5% of women will experience 2 consecutive losses, and only 1% will experience 3 or more.[1]

RPL is often idiopathic. Of the 50% of cases that have a discernible cause, most are attributable to the following factors:

- Anatomic (congenital or acquired uterine abnormalities, including a septate, unicornuate, or didelphic uterus; submucosal fibroid; or intrauterine synechiae)
- Endocrine (thyroid disorders, hyperprolactinemia, diabetes mellitus)
- Immunologic (antiphospholipid antibody syndrome)
- Genetic (aneuploidy, structural rearrangements)
- Other (infectious, environmental)

This review focuses on the genetic causes of RPL, along with the appropriate workup of products of conception (POC), and management options, including expectant management (EM) and in vitro fertilization (IVF) with preimplantation genetic screening (PGS).

OVERVIEW OF THE GENETIC CAUSES OF RECURRENT PREGNANCY LOSS

Pregnancy loss can occur because of numerical chromosomal abnormalities, arising from meiotic nondisjunction (eg, trisomy or monosomy), aberrant fertilization (eg, triploidy), or embryogenesis (eg, tetraploidy), or because of structural chromosomal abnormalities, arising from the inheritance of a derivative chromosome (eg, translocations and inversions). Estimates of the incidence and outcome of various karyotypic abnormalities are shown in **Table 1**.[2]

Table 1 Estimated incidence and outcome of various karyotypic abnormalities in 10,000 pregnancies			
	Incidence per 10,000 Pregnancies	Spontaneous Abortion (%)	Live Births
Total	10,000	1500 (15)	8500
Normal chromosomes	9200	750 (8)	8450
Abnormal chromosomes	800	750 (94)	50
Specific abnormalities			
Polyploid	170	170 (100)	0
45,X	140	139 (99)	1
Trisomy 16	112	112 (100)	0
Trisomy 18	20	19 (95)	1
Trisomy 21	45	35 (78)	10
Trisomy, other	209	208 (99.5)	1
47,XXY; 47,XXX; 47,XYY	19	4 (21)	15
Unbalanced rearrangement	27	23 (85)	4
Balanced rearrangement	19	3 (16)	16
Other	39	37 (95)	2

These estimates are based on observed frequencies of chromosome abnormalities in miscarriage specimens and live-born infants. It is possible that the frequency of these abnormalities is much higher, though, because many spontaneously abort before clinical recognition.
Adapted from Nussbaum RL, McInnes RR, Willard HF. Principles of clinical cytogenetics and genome analysis. In: Nussbaum RL, McInnes RR, Willard HF, editors. Thompson & Thompson genetics in medicine. 8th edition. Philadelphia: Elsevier; 2016. p. 73; with permission.

Numerical Chromosomal Abnormalities

Miscarriage is overwhelmingly due to numerical chromosomal abnormalities, with the gain or loss of a whole chromosome or the presence of an abnormal chromosomal complement (3n or 4n). An early cytogenetic study of 1500 miscarriage specimens reported that more than 61% of samples contained an abnormal karyotype, including trisomy, monosomy, triploidy, or tetraploidy.[3] The single most common chromosomal abnormality was 45,X; the single most common class of abnormalities was trisomy, with trisomy 16 and 22 the most frequently observed. Of note, when stratified according to female age, the distribution of cytogenetic abnormalities is similar between patients with RPL and sporadic miscarriage.[4] As described further in later discussion, such analyses that rely on conventional metaphase karyotyping with Giemsa staining (ie, G-banding) may actually underestimate the proportion of abnormal samples as a result of culture failure and false negatives from maternal cell contamination (MCC).

Although other mechanisms such as recombination failure and premature separation of homologs or sister chromatids exist, meiotic nondisjunction is the most common cause of aneuploidy.[5] Meiotic nondisjunction refers to the failure of a chromosome pair to segregate properly during 1 of the 2 meiotic divisions, which results in disomic or nullisomic gametes. Fertilization of such gamete produces either a trisomic or a monosomic zygote, respectively. Postmeiotic, or mitotic, nondisjunction can also occur, which results in mosaicism with clonal expansion of multiple cell lines. The timing of these errors, along with the resulting abnormal genotypes, is depicted graphically in **Fig. 1**.

Most human aneuploidies are maternally derived and increase as a function of female age.[5] It has been estimated that only 7% of fetal trisomies arise from paternal meiotic errors.[6] The reason for this notable sexual dimorphism in error rates is not fully understood, but may be explained by the following 2 observations: (1) spermatocytes with synaptic defects in the pachytene stage of prophase I or metaphase I typically undergo apoptosis, whereas oocytes with similar defects remain viable; and (2) although spermatogenesis is a continuous process, oogenesis is not, such that oocytes arrested in prophase I have a disproportionate amount of time from birth until ovulation to incur genetic insults, including disturbances to the synaptonemal complex

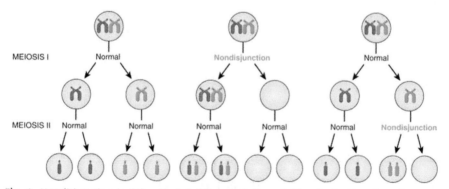

Fig. 1. Nondisjunction in (*A*) meiosis I, (*B*) meiosis II, and (*C*) mitosis. Note how improper chromosomal segregation in meiosis results in nullisomic and disomic gametes, and similar events in mitosis result in clonal populations of mosaic cell lines. (*From* Nussbaum RL, McInnes RR, Willard HF. Principles of clinical cytogenetics and genome analysis. In: Nussbaum RL, McInnes RR, Willard HF, et al, editors. Thompson & Thompson Genetics in Medicine. 8th edition. Philadelphia: Elsevier; 2016:57–74; with permission.)

and loss of cohesion between homologs and sister chromatids.[7] Indeed, the frequency and placement of crossovers, which are necessary to maintain synapsis in prophase I, are strongly associated with the propensity of a chromosome pair to segregate properly. Three abnormal configurations, in particular, predispose to numerical chromosome abnormalities: absent crossovers (otherwise known as achiasmate bivalents), distal-only or telomeric crossovers, and proximal or centromeric crossovers.[5] Furthermore, loss of cohesion between homologs in anaphase I and sister chromatids in anaphase II likely also contributes to the increasing frequency of chromosomal segregation errors in the aging oocyte.

Patients undergoing IVF with PGS provide an informative model for examining the effect of female age on aneuploidy rates. Franasiak and colleagues[8] examined the PGS results from 15,169 consecutive embryos biopsied at the blastocyst stage contributed by 2701 patients. The frequency of aneuploid embryos as a function of female age is striking, as shown in **Fig. 2**. Among the 6168 aneuploid samples, errors involving a single chromosome were the most commonly observed (63.7%), followed by 2 chromosomes (19.9%) and 3 or more chromosomes (16.3%). The likelihood of an embryo being called complex abnormal (ie, having 3 or more numerical chromosome abnormalities) was significantly associated with increasing female age. Interestingly, the rate of aneuploidy was likewise associated with chromosomal structure: acrocentric chromosomes exhibited the highest aneuploidy rates, followed by metacentric chromosomes, and finally, submetacentric chromosomes.[9]

Structural Chromosomal Abnormalities

Chromosomal rearrangements can also lead to the production of unbalanced gametes. There are various types of structural anomalies associated with RPL, including

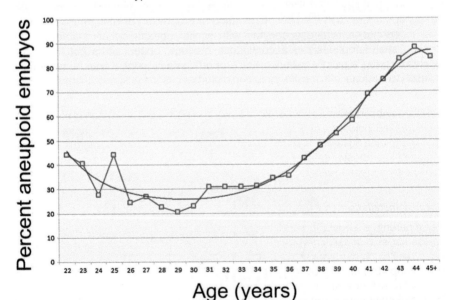

Fig. 2. Prevalence of embryonic aneuploidy relative to female age in a general infertility population (n = 2701 patients; 15,169 blastocysts) undergoing PGS with quantitative PCR. (*From* Franasiak JM, Forman EJ, Hong KH, et al. The nature of aneuploidy with increasing age of the female partner: a review of 15,169 consecutive trophectoderm biopsies evaluated with comprehensive chromosomal screening. Fertil Steril 2014;101(3):660; with permission.)

translocations, inversions, insertions, and ring chromosomes (**Fig. 3**). It is estimated that 2% to 5% of couples with RPL have a structural chromosomal abnormality, as opposed to 0.2% of the general population.[10,11] Like the numerical abnormalities, structural rearrangements may be present in all cells or may be mosaic in nature. The reproductive risk due to structural abnormalities depends on the type of rearrangement and whether the male or female partner is the carrier.[12,13]

Translocations
A translocation involves the exchange of chromosomal segments between 2 chromosomes and can be classified as reciprocal or Robertsonian.[2] In the RPL population, reciprocal translocations are the most common structural abnormality found. In a series of 51 couples with RPL and a documented structural rearrangement, 28/51 (54.9%) had a reciprocal translocation and 12/51 (23.5%) had a Robertsonian one.[4]

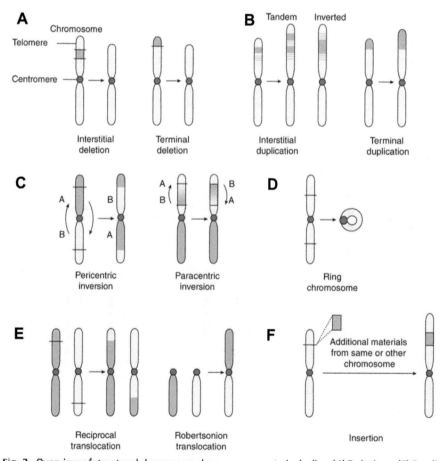

Fig. 3. Overview of structural chromosomal rearrangements, including (*A*) Deletions, (*B*) Duplications, (*C*) Ring chromosomes, (*D*) Isochromosomes, (*E*) Robertsonian translocations, and (*F*) Reciprocal translocations. (*From* Nussbaum RL, McInnes RR, Willard HF. Principles of clinical cytogenetics and genome analysis. In: Nussbaum RL, McInnes RR, Willard HF, et al, editors. Thompson & Thompson Genetics in Medicine, 8th edition. Philadelphia: Elsevier; 2016. p. 68; with permission.)

Reciprocal translocations occur when 2 chromosomes exchange segments via double-strand breakage with nonhomologous end joining or via recombination. Provided that the exchange is truly reciprocal with no loss or gain of chromosomal material, and the breakpoint does not involve a critical gene, typically reciprocal translocation carriers are phenotypically normal.[2] Patients with such rearrangements have an increased risk of RPL, though, because of the production of unbalanced gametes. During meiosis, a quadrivalent is necessary to ensure proper alignment of the 2 derivative chromosomes and the 2 normal chromosomes. Depending on how the members of the quadrivalent segregate to opposite poles (alternate, adjacent-1, or adjacent-2), normal, balanced, and unbalanced gametes will result.[2] As shown in **Fig. 4**, alternate segregation produces normal and balanced gametes, whereas the adjacent patterns always yield unbalanced gametes.

Robertsonian translocations occur when 2 acrocentric chromosomes (13, 14, 15, 21, and 22) break or recombine, with the long arms fusing at the centromere to form a derivative chromosome, and the short arms fusing at the centromere to form a separate derivative chromosome. With subsequent cell divisions, the short-arm rearrangement is lost. Because the short arms in these acrocentric chromosomes only contain nonessential satellite DNA and ribosomal RNA genes, there is typically no associated phenotype.[2] As opposed to the quadrivalent formation in meiosis among balanced translocation carriers, a trivalent is formed among Robertsonian translocation carriers. Similarly, segregation patterns inform whether balanced or unbalanced gametes are produced. Of note, the likelihood of a viable, unbalanced gestation is

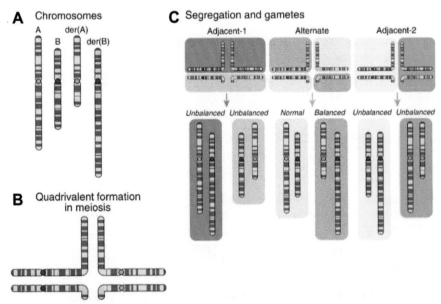

Fig. 4. (*A*) Balanced translocation with resulting derivative chromosomes. (*B*) During meiosis, quadrivalent formation is necessary to allow proper alignment between the normal and derivative chromosomes. (*C*) Segregation patterns (adjacent-1, alternate, and adjacent-2) in a translocation carrier with resulting normal, balanced, or unbalanced gametes. (*From* Nussbaum RL, McInnes RR, Willard HF. Principles of clinical cytogenetics and genome analysis. In: Nussbaum RL, McInnes RR, Willard HF, editors. Thompson & Thompson genetics in medicine. 8th edition. Philadelphia: Elsevier; 2016. p. 70; with permission.)

related to whether the female or male partner is the translocation carrier[12]; in the case of a Robertsonian translocation involving chromosome 21, for example, the risk is significantly higher if the translocation is of maternal origin (15% vs 0.5%).[13]

Inversions

An inversion involves 2 double-strand break points within a single chromosome, with subsequent reversal of the intervening segment.[2] Inversions can be paracentric (in one arm of a chromosome) or pericentric (involving the centromere, and therefore both arms). An inversion is another type of balanced rearrangement that does not have an associated phenotype, but can lead to unbalanced gametes because a loop is necessary to allow proper chromosomal alignment during meiosis, and recombination can occur within this loop. The unbalanced gamete from a paracentric inversion will not be viable because it will be acentric or dicentric; in contrast, the unbalanced gamete from a pericentric inversion can be viable, with resulting duplication or loss of chromosomal segments (ie, leading to partial trisomy or partial monosomy).[14] In one series of couples with RPL, 7/51 (13.7%) patients with a documented structural rearrangement carried an inversion.[4]

Other rearrangements

Other structural chromosomal abnormalities are possible and may be rarely found in patients with RPL, including ring chromosomes, insertions, and complex rearrangements involving 3 or more breakpoints. In a series of 51 couples with RPL and documented karyotypic abnormalities, 1/51 (2%) had a ring chromosome and 3/51 (5.9%) harbored an insertion.[4]

Single Nucleotide Polymorphisms and Copy Number Variants Associated with Recurrent Pregnancy Loss

Molecular techniques, such as single nucleotide polymorphism (SNP) microarray, array comparative genomic hybridization (CGH), and next-generation sequencing, have revealed possible candidate genes associated with RPL. Most of these genes have been described in only small case-control studies. Examples of SNPs and copy number variants (CNVs) that may contribute to a genetic susceptibility to miscarriage include variances in the following genes: *AR, DNMT3, FOXP3, CGB5, NLRP7, TIMP2,* and *CTNNA3*.[15–20]

A recent systematic review of 428 case-control studies from 1990 to 2015 evaluated 472 variants in 187 genes.[21] Meta-analysis could only be performed for 36 variants in 16 genes, because the other studies had never been replicated. The investigators reported modest associations between RPL and 21 variants in genes (odds ratio [OR] 0.51–2.37) involved in the immune response (*IFNG, IL10, KIR2DS2, KIR2DS3, KIR2DS4, MBL, TNF*), coagulation (*F2, F5, PAI-1, PROZ*), metabolism (*GSTT1, MTHFR*), and angiogenesis (*NOS3, VEGFA*). The epidemiologic data credibility was deemed to be weak to moderate. Although future investigation will assuredly clarify whether these and other variants do indeed modify the risk of miscarriage, clinical application of these putative variants in the RPL population is not advised at the present time outside of research protocols.

Of note, despite the associations noted above, mutations in the thrombophilia genes, including *MTHFR, F2,* and *F5*, and deficiencies in protein C, protein S, and antithrombin III, may increase the risk of second- or third-trimester loss, but current evidence does not support routine testing or treatment of these conditions in the RPL population in the absence of other risk factors like a personal or family history of venous thromboembolism.[22]

EVALUATION OF PRODUCTS OF CONCEPTION

Traditionally, miscarriage specimens were evaluated by conventional metaphase karyotyping using G-banding with a resolution of approximately 10 Mb. This technique has notable limitations, including the requirement for cell culture, high culture failure rate (10%–40%), labor intensity, inability to detect submicroscopic deletions and duplications of clinical significance, and the possibility of false negative results due to MCC.[23]

Newer molecular techniques like SNP microarray or array comparative genomic hybridization offer several advantages. First, no cell culture is required, which avoids culture failure, contamination, overgrowth with maternal cells, and selection against mosaic cell lines.[24] Second, test results are typically available in a shorter amount of time and are not dependent on user variability, but rather the bioinformatics packages applied. Third, these techniques provide much higher resolution and allow detection of microduplications and microdeletions below the traditional 10-Mb resolution of G-banding. The clinical relevance of this higher-resolution platform was demonstrated in an analysis of 755 samples determined to be normal by conventional karyotyping that were reevaluated by SNP array.[25] In this series, 33/775 (4.4%) had a CNV ranging in size from 400 Kb to 9.5 Mb. Twelve of 33 (36.4%, or 1.6% of those called normal by G-banding) were classified as clinically significant, whereas the remainders were considered variants of unknown significance. Furthermore, 3/755 (0.4%) of cases considered normal at the G-band level were determined to have uniparental disomy. A fourth advantage of array-based platforms is that they allow detection of MCC; indeed, SNP array identified MCC in 528/2392 (22.1%) miscarriage specimens. This could lead to an underrepresentation of abnormalities called by karyotyping. Fifth, these techniques can be applied to archival tissue from prior miscarriages stored in formaldehyde-fixed, paraffin-embedded blocks. Such "rescue karyotyping" can thus be performed on curettage specimens that were never sent for karyotypic analysis or to allow reanalysis of specimens that were called normal by conventional G-banding.[26] Sixth, in the case of SNP array, the parental origin of aneuploidy can be determined.

It should be noted that aCGH cannot detect balanced translocations, whereas SNP arrays can provided that parental DNA is available to phase the reciprocal translocation carrier. aCGH also requires short tandem repeat (STR) microsatellite analysis to detect MCC and some polyploidy,[23] whereas SNP array is unable to detect balanced tetraploidy.

The first head-to-head comparison of conventional cytogenetics, aCGH, and SNP array for POC analysis was recently reported.[23] Shah and colleagues[23] performed a prospective blinded study of 60 miscarriages from first-trimester curettage specimens; chorionic villi were separated equally for concurrent analysis using the 3 techniques. A correct call was defined as a result that was concordant between any 2 testing platforms, and the correct call rate was similar for the various techniques (cytogenetics: 85%; aCGH: 85%; SNP: 93%). Discordant calls were due to MCC, balanced rearrangements, polyploidy, and mosaicism. Of note, this study did not uniformly apply STR analysis to the aCGH platform. The kappa statistic for interrater agreement was 0.65, indicating substantial agreement. There were 4 cases of culture failure (7%), and 6 of the remaining 56 samples (11%) were inconclusive because of a 46,XX result that could not distinguish between normal fetal female karyotype and MCC without subsequent molecular testing. The investigators conclude that each method of analysis contains inherent limitations and offers similar performance characteristics; thus, providers may choose the method of analysis based on local availability and consideration of these limitations with respect to the specific clinical scenario.[23] The cost-efficacy of these various platforms for POC analysis has never been compared.

MANAGEMENT OPTIONS FOR GENETIC CAUSES OF RECURRENT PREGNANCY LOSS

Management of RPL depends on the identified cause. For couples with recurrent aneuploidy or unbalanced losses, the available options include EM or IVF/PGS/preimplantation genetic diagnosis (PGD). There are limited data available comparing these 2 treatment strategies in the RPL population. In a retrospective cohort study of RPL patients with structural chromosomal rearrangements, the use of PGD was associated with a significant reduction in the number of miscarriages before live birth ($P = .02$), but no difference in cumulative live birth rates (PGD: 25/37, 67.6% vs EM: 34/52, 65.2%; OR 1.10, 95% confidence interval 0.45–2.70; $P = .83$).[27] Subsequent retrospective analyses among RPL patients *without* structural rearrangements likewise demonstrated a trend toward decreased clinical miscarriage rates in the group transferring a euploid embryo (14% vs 24%; $P = .12$) and a significant increase in live birth rate for the subgroup of patients older than age 35 years who elected PGS and underwent a euploid transfer (59% vs 28%; $P = .0001$).[28] These investigators then performed an intention-to-treat (ITT) analysis of the same data, in which they determined the live birth rate per attempt number; for the PGS group, an attempt was defined on a per-cycle start basis, and for the EM group, an attempt was defined as 6 calendar months. When analyzed according to ITT in this manner, there were no differences in live birth rate (PGS: 63/198, 32% vs EM: 68/202, 34%; $P = .75$) or miscarriage rate (PGS: 18/198, 20% vs EM: 25/202, 24%; $P = .61$). Although such an analysis incorporates PGS cycles in which embryo biopsy was canceled due to poor development and embryo transfer was canceled due to no euploid embryo available, it also illustrates why an ITT analysis should not be performed on retrospective data. First, no randomization was performed and selection bias is apparent based on the 2-year difference in mean patient age (PGS: 37.1 ± 4.1 vs EM: 35.7 ± 3.9 years; $P = .004$). Such a difference may have a profound impact on the expected rate of aneuploidy. Second, approximately 20% (40/198) of the planned blastocyst stage PGS cycles were canceled because of poor embryo development and were converted to cleavage stage transfer without PGS. The ITT principle requires analysis of outcomes according to the initial allocation; here, the planned PGS cycle was canceled in favor of an unbiopsied day 3 embryo transfer, which was not the other intervention that was analyzed in this study (6 months of EM). Similarly, patients in the EM group were not included if they crossed over to the PGS group part way through an attempt; as a result, only the experimental group was subject to an intervention that was different than its initial allocation. Furthermore, results are informed by the definition of attempt for EM and may be appreciably different if attempt was defined as 3 or 9 months of trying, for example. Thus, to define post hoc what the unit of analysis is and then compare outcomes between mutually exclusive interventions undermines the ITT principle and underscores why such analyses should only be performed in randomized studies.

Indeed, high-quality data regarding the role of PGS in the RPL population are lacking. In decision analytical models, PGS is more costly per live birth than EM.[29] The physical, emotional, and financial burden of experiencing another miscarriage for an RPL patient, though, is difficult to assess and may vary from couple to couple. Accordingly, how does one assign a value to the prevention of such a loss? Most would agree that if it were possible to prevent another miscarriage through some intervention, as long the intervention posed minimal risk, then couples with RPL would likely readily pursue treatment.

An appropriately designed study evaluating the preferred management strategy for RPL patients has yet to be performed. The ideal study would randomize patients with RPL (≥2 clinical losses with sonographic or pathologic confirmation) to EM or IVF with blastocyst biopsy, molecular analysis using a contemporary PGS platform, and planned frozen embryo transfer. Randomization would be blocked on idiopathic RPL versus carriers of a structural chromosomal rearrangement. Rather than defining success by the time spent in treatment or cumulative live birth rate, which are often metrics used in the general infertility population, a more meaningful primary endpoint for RPL patients would be a survival analysis of the number of miscarriages before establishing an ongoing viable pregnancy. Secondary endpoints would include the time spent in treatment, cumulative live birth rates, and associated medical costs. This design would also allow calculation of attrition rates for each group. Standardized questionnaires would be collected to assess the burden of care in each group. Until such a study is completed, though, questions will remain among patients and physicians alike about the preferred management of RPL due to recurrent aneuploidy or structural chromosomal rearrangements.

SUMMARY

In conclusion, numerical and structural chromosomal abnormalities are important causes of RPL. Most miscarriages are aneuploid in nature, and the rate and complexity of aneuploidy are driven primarily by female age. Balanced translocations or inversions can lead to unbalanced gametes depending on specific recombination and segregation patterns (alternate, adjacent-1, and adjacent-2) during meiosis. The attendant reproductive risk depends on the type of rearrangement and its parental origin.

Current methods for POC analysis include cytogenetics, array CGH, and SNP microarray. The performance characteristics and interrater agreement of these techniques are similar, and each platform has its respective advantages and disadvantages. Specifically, although conventional G-banding is the gold standard for chromosomal rearrangement and detection of polyploidy, it is subject to important limitations, including culture failure, turnaround time, false negatives due to MCC, and low resolution that does not allow detection of microduplications or microdeletions or uniparental disomy. Molecular platforms offer quicker results without the need for cell culture, higher resolution that allows detection of submicroscopic abnormalities, discrimination between fetal 46,XX and MCC, processing of archival tissue from paraffin blocks, and determination of the parental origin of aneuploidy.

The preferred treatment strategy (EM vs PGS) remains a matter of active research. PGS with selection and transfer of a euploid embryo has been shown to significantly decrease the risk of subsequent miscarriage, but further investigation of this emerging strategy is needed before routine adoption in the RPL population.

REFERENCES

1. Rai R. Recurrent miscarriage. Lancet 2006;368:601–11.
2. Nussbaum RL, McInnes RR, Willard HF. Principles of clinical cytogenetics and genome analysis. In: Thompson Thompson, editor. Genetics in medicine. 8th edition. Philadelphia: Elsevier; 2016. p. 57–74.
3. Boue J, Boue A, Lazar P. Retrospective and prospective epidemiological studies of 1500 karyotyped spontaneous human abortions. Teratology 1975;12:11–26.
4. Stephenson MD, Awartani KA, Robinson WP. Cytogenetic analysis of miscarriages from couples with recurrent miscarriage: a case-control study. Hum Reprod 2002;17:446–51.
5. Nussbaum RL, McInnes RR, Willard HF. Principles of clinical cytogenetics and genome analysis. In: Nussbaum RL, McInnes RR, Willard HF, et al, editors.

Thompson & Thompson Genetics in Medicine. 8th edition. Philadelphia: Elsevier; 2016. p. 57–74.

6. Robinson WP, Bernasconi F, Lau A, et al. Frequency of meiotic trisomy depends on involved chromosome and mode of ascertainment. Am J Med Genet 1999;84:34–42.

7. Hunt PA, Hassold TJ. Sex matters in meiosis. Science 2002;296:2181–3.

8. Franasiak JM, Forman EJ, Hong KH, et al. The nature of aneuploidy with increasing age of the female partner: a review of 15,169 consecutive trophecto-derm biopsies evaluated with comprehensive chromosomal screening. Fertil Steril 2014;101:656–63.

9. Franasiak JM, Forman EJ, Hong KH, et al. Aneuploidy across individual chromosomes at the embryonic level in trophectoderm biopsies: changes with patient age and chromosome structure. J Assist Reprod Genet 2014;31:1501–9.

10. Jacobs PA, Brown C, Gregson N, et al. Estimates of the frequency of chromosome abnormalities detectable in unselected newborns using moderate levels of banding. J Med Genet 1992;29:103–8.

11. De Braekeleer M, Dao TN. Cytogenetic studies in couples experiencing repeated pregnancy losses. Hum Reprod 1990;5:519–28.

12. Munne S, Escudero T, Sandalinas M, et al. Gamete segregation in female carriers of Robertsonian translocations. Cytogenet Cell Genet 2000;90:303–8.

13. Boue A, Gallano P. A collaborative study of the segregation of inherited chromosome structural rearrangements in 1356 prenatal diagnoses. Prenat Diagn 1984; 4:45–67.

14. Morin SJ, Eccles J, Iturriaga A, et al. Translocations, inversions and other chromosome rearrangements. Fertil Steril 2017;107:19–26.

15. Porras-Dorantes Á, Brambila-Tapia AJL, Lazcano-Castellanos AB, et al. Association between G1733A (rs6152) polymorphism in androgen receptor gene and recurrent spontaneous abortions in Mexican population. J Assist Reprod Genet 2017. https://doi.org/10.1007/s10815-017-0993-4.

16. Liu Y, Zheng H, Guo P, et al. DNA methyltransferase 3A promoter polymorphism is associated with the risk of human spontaneous abortion after assisted reproduction techniques and natural conception. J Assist Reprod Genet 2017;34:245–52.

17. Saxena D, Misra MK, Parveen F, et al. The transcription factor Forkhead Box P3 gene variants affect idiopathic recurrent pregnancy loss. Placenta 2015;36: 226–31.

18. Sun Y, Ji X. Association of rs7260002 of chorionic gonadotrophin β5 with idiopathic recurrent spontaneous abortion in Chinese population. J Assist Reprod Genet 2014;31:1497–500.

19. Huang JY, Su M, Lin SH, et al. A genetic association study of NLRP2 and NLRP7 genes in idiopathic recurrent miscarriage. Hum Reprod 2013;28:1127–34.

20. Rajcan-Separovic E, Diego-Alvarez D, Robinson WP, et al. Identification of copy number variants in miscarriages from couples with idiopathic recurrent pregnancy loss. Hum Reprod 2010;25:2913–22.

21. Pereza N, Ostojic S, Kapovic M, et al. Systematic review and meta-analysis of genetic association studies in idiopathic recurrent spontaneous abortion. Fertil Steril 2017;107:150–9.

22. De Jong PG, Goddijin M, Middwldorp S. Testing for inherited thrombophilia in recurrent miscarriage. Semin Reprod Med 2011;29:540–5.

23. Shah MS, Cinnioglu C, Maisenbacher M, et al. Comparison of cytogenetics and molecular karyotyping for chromosome testing of miscarriage specimens. Fertil Steril 2017;104:1028–33.

24. Robberecht C, Schuddinck V, Fryns JP, et al. Diagnosis of miscarriages by molecular karyotyping: benefits and pitfalls. Genet Med 2009;11:646–54.
25. Levy B, Sigurjonsson S, Pettersen B, et al. Genomic imbalance in products of conception: single nucleotide polymorphism chromosomal microarray analysis. Obstet Gynecol 2014;124:202–9.
26. Kudesia R, Li M, Smith J, et al. Rescue karyotyping: a case series of array-based comparative genomic hybridization evaluation of archival conceptual tissue. Reprod Biol Endocrinol 2014;14:19.
27. Ikuma S, Sato T, Sugiura-Ogasawara M, et al. Preimplantation genetic diagnosis and natural conception: a comparison of live birth rates in patients with recurrent pregnancy loss associated with translocation. PLoS One 2015;10:e0129958.
28. Murugappan G, Shahine LK, Perfetto CO, et al. Intent to treat analysis of in vitro fertilization and preimplantation genetic screening versus expectant management in patients with recurrent pregnancy loss. Hum Reprod 2016;31:1668–74.
29. Murugappan G, Ohno MS, Lathi RB. Cost-effectiveness analysis of preimplantation genetic screening and in vitro fertilization versus expectant management in patients with unexplained recurrent pregnancy loss. Fertil Steril 2015;103: 1215–20.

Hereditary Cancers in Gynecology

What Physicians Should Know About Genetic Testing, Screening, and Risk Reduction

Kari L. Ring, MD, MS*, Susan C. Modesitt, MD

KEYWORDS

- Hereditary cancer syndrome • BRCA • Lynch syndrome • Screening
- Risk reduction

KEY POINTS

- A thorough family history should be taken and updated during annual gynecologic care.
- There are well-described situations that might herald the need for referral to a genetic or high-risk specialist for further evaluation.
- Clinicians must take the mutation of interest, the personal history, and the family history into consideration when designing a personalized screening and risk-reduction strategy for each individual patient.

INTRODUCTION

All cancer is genetic. That is to say that cancer cells carry somatic genetic mutations/alterations that cause unregulated growth of the cancer's cells and the ability to metastasize. Yet, most cancers are not hereditary, in the sense that women are born with a genetic predisposition/genetic mutation that specifically caused their cancer. As essentially primary care physicians for women, obstetrician gynecologists (OB/GYN) must be able to recognize the women in their practices who might harbor a genetic predisposition to cancer so that they can institute proven screening and risk-reduction measures for their patient and her extended family as appropriate. Although phenomenal progress has been made in cancer treatment with the advent of newer chemotherapeutic regimens, targeted therapies, and immunotherapy, cures for malignancies are simply not guaranteed and thus, primary prevention of cancers rather than treatment should remain the gold standard when applicable.

Conflict of Interest Statement: The authors report no conflict of interest.
Division of Gynecologic Oncology, Department of Obstetrics and Gynecology, University of Virginia Health System, Box 800712, Charlottesville, VA 22908-0712, USA
* Corresponding author.
E-mail address: KEL7J@hscmail.mcc.virginia.edu

Obstet Gynecol Clin N Am 45 (2018) 155–173
https://doi.org/10.1016/j.ogc.2017.10.011
0889-8545/18/© 2017 Elsevier Inc. All rights reserved.

obgyn.theclinics.com

Hereditary cancer knowledge has grown exponentially in recent years since the elucidation of the human genome; this increased understanding of genetic cancer predisposition must translate into better identification of at-risk women by OB/GYN practitioners with appropriate evaluation by cancer genetics experts for coordination of genetic testing, cancer screening, and risk-reduction measures. This article presents general guidelines and potential tools for identification of high-risk patients, reviews the current literature regarding genetic mutations associated with gynecologic malignancies, and proposes screening and risk-reduction options for high-risk patients.

HEREDITARY CANCER SYNDROMES

Although all of the genes discussed carry a significantly increased lifetime risk of developing gynecologic malignancies, their associated cancer risks, even for individual genes within a syndrome, are not equivalent. It is essential that clinicians consider the mutation of interest, personal history of cancers, and family history of cancers in concert when counseling patients and outlining risk-reduction strategies.

Hereditary Breast and Ovarian Cancer

Mutations in BRCA1 and BRCA2 place patients at an increased lifetime risk of multiple cancers, most notably breast and ovarian cancer (**Box 1**). Germline mutations in BRCA1 and BRCA2 account for most hereditary ovarian cancers and mutations in these genes may account for up to 18% of all ovarian cancers.[1] These mutations are inherited in an autosomal-dominant fashion. BRCA1 and BRCA2 carry similar lifetime risks of breast cancer of 80%; however, women who harbor a germline mutation in BRCA1 have a higher lifetime risk of developing ovarian cancer compared with BRCA2 mutation carriers, with a cumulative lifetime risk of 39% to 46% and 11% to 27%, respectively.[2–4] In addition, BRCA1-associated breast and ovarian cancers present at an earlier age compared with BRCA2-associated cancers; BRCA1 mutation carriers present about a decade earlier than their BRCA2 counterparts.[4] Given the

---

Box 1
Common hereditary cancer syndromes encountered by obstetrician gynecologists and associated clinical features: hereditary breast/ovarian cancer

Associated mutations
• BRCA 1 and BRCA2

Hallmark family history components[a]
• Multiple generations affected by breast cancer (or related cancers) at younger ages
• Any male breast cancer diagnosis
• Any ovarian cancer diagnosis
• Triple negative breast cancer in a woman at 60 years of age or less
• Pancreatic cancer in combination with other cancers
• Ashkenazi Jewish

Associated cancers
• Breast cancer
• Ovarian cancer
• Pancreatic cancer
• Melanoma
• Aggressive prostate cancer

[a] Not all families meet every criteria but any of these should be explored for a possible link to hereditary breast and ovarian cancer.
Data from Refs.[6,14,32]

increasing proportion of ovarian cancers associated with *BRCA* mutations, the Society for Gynecologic Oncology (SGO) released a clinical practice statement in 2014 that recommends physicians offer genetic testing for *BRCA1* and *BRCA2* in all newly diagnosed epithelial ovarian, tubal, and primary peritoneal cancers.[5] This recommendation was later endorsed by the National Comprehensive Cancer network (NCCN).[6] In addition to breast and ovarian cancer, *BRCA* mutation carriers are also at an increased risk of other cancers including pancreatic cancer, melanoma, and potentially uterine cancer for *BRCA1* mutation carriers (**Table 1**).[7–9]

Hereditary Ovarian Cancer

BRCA1 and *BRCA2* function in the homologous recombination pathway, which is responsible for DNA double-strand repair. Other genes that function in this pathway have also been recently associated with an increased lifetime risk of ovarian cancer, including *RAD51C*, *RAD51D*, and *BRIP1*. Mutations in these moderate penetrance genes place patients at a lifetime risk of ovarian cancer of 10% (see **Table 1**).[10–12] It should be noted that these genes have not as of yet been associated with an increased lifetime risk of breast cancer. In addition, other genes within the DNA double-strand repair pathway, including *PALB2* and *BARD1*, have been evaluated, but to date have not been shown to significantly increase the risk of ovarian cancer.

Lynch Syndrome

Germline mutations in one of the four mismatch repair (MMR) proteins (*MLH1*, *MSH2*, *MSH6*, and *PMS2*) or *EPCAM*, the regulator of *MSH2*, account for 15% of all hereditary cancers and are inherited in an autosomal-dominant fashion (**Box 2**). Patients with Lynch syndrome are at an increased lifetime risk of multiple cancers including colorectal cancer, endometrial cancer, ovarian cancer, gastric cancer, small bowel cancer, transitional cell carcinoma of the genitourinary tract, pancreatic cancer, sebaceous adenomas, and glioblastoma multiforme (see **Table 1**).[13,14] In terms of gynecologic cancers, endometrial cancer is the most common type of malignancy and accounts for 2% to 6% of all endometrial cancers.[15] Indeed, women with Lynch syndrome are more likely to present with a gynecologic cancer, such as endometrial or ovarian cancer, rather than a colon cancer, emphasizing the importance of OB/GYNs in the identification of these patients.[16] Lynch-associated ovarian cancers tend to present at a young age and are more likely to be of endometrioid or clear cell histology.[17,18] Lynch syndrome is a unique hereditary cancer syndrome because the specific tumors can be tested for markers of microsatellite instability to identify patients that may carry a germline mutation. Immunohistochemistry (IHC) for the four Lynch proteins (*MLH1*, *MSH2*, *MSH6*, and *PMS2*) and polymerase chain reaction–based microsatellite instability analysis can be performed on tumors to help guide germline testing. It should be noted that a proportion of endometrial cancers have loss of expression of *MLH1* on tumor testing caused by sporadic promoter methylation. Thus, if IHC is used as a screening technique, *MLH1* methylation analysis should be applied to all tumors with loss of *MLH1* expression because these are not caused by a germline mutation. Consistent with colorectal recommendations, the SGO released a clinical practice statement in 2014 recommending systematic screening for Lynch syndrome in all newly diagnosed endometrial cancers.[19]

Polymerase Proofreading Associated Polyposis

Recently, mutations in two genes that function in conjunction with the Lynch syndrome complex, *POLD1* and *POLE*, have been associated with an increased risk of malignancy, similar to Lynch syndrome, and are inherited in an autosomal-dominant

Table 1
Hereditary gynecologic syndromes and associated cancer risks

Gene	Genetic Syndrome	Cancer Type	Cancer Risk (%)[6,10–12,14,30]
BRCA1	HBOC	Ovary	39–46
		Breast	65–85
BRCA2	HBOC	Ovary	10–27
		Breast	45–85
		Pancreas	Elevated[a]
		Melanoma	Elevated[a]
BRIP1	HOC	Ovary	10–15
RAD51C	HOC	Ovary	10–15
RAD51D	HOC	Ovary	10–15
MLH1	LS	Uterus	25–60
		Ovary	4–24
		Colon	52–82
		Gastric	6–13
		Hepatobiliary tract	1–4
		Small bowel	3–6
		Urothelial	1–7
		CNS	1–3
		Pancreatic	1–6
		Sebaceous neoplasms	1–9
MSH2/EPCAM	LS	Uterus	25–60
		Ovary	4–24
		Colon	52–82
		Gastric	6–13
		Hepatobiliary tract	1–4
		Small bowel	3–6
		Urothelial	1–7
		CNS	1–3
		Pancreatic	1–6
		Sebaceous neoplasms	1–6
MSH6	LS	Uterus	16–26
		Ovary	1–11
		Colon	10–22
		Gastric	≤3
		Hepatobiliary tract	NR
		Small bowel	NR
		Urothelial	<1
		CNS	NR
		Pancreatic	NR
PMS2	LS	Uterus	15
		Ovary	6[b]
		Colon	15–20
		Gastric	6[b]
		Hepatobiliary tract	6[b]
		Small bowel	6[b]
		Urothelial	6[b]
		CNS	6[b]
		Pancreatic	NR
		Sebaceous neoplasms	NR
POLD1	PPAP	Uterus	Elevated[a]
		Colon	Elevated[a]

(continued on next page)

Table 1
(*continued*)

Gene	Genetic Syndrome	Cancer Type	Cancer Risk (%)[6,10–12,14,30]
PTEN	Cowden	Uterus	19–28
		Breast	25–50
		Follicular thyroid	3–38
		Renal cell	2–5
		Colon	9
STK11/LKB1	PJS	Ovary (SCTAT)	18–21
		Uterus	9
		Cervix (adenoma malignum)	10
		Breast	45–50
		Colon	39
		Gastric	29
		Small intestine	13
		Pancreas	11–36
		Lung	15–17
TP53	Li-Fraumeni	Ovary	Elevated[a]
		Uterus	Elevated[a]
		Breast	Elevated[c]
		CNS	Elevated[c]
		Soft tissue sarcoma	Elevated[c]
		Bone sarcoma	Elevated[c]
		Adrenocortical carcinoma	Elevated[c]
		Leukemia	Elevated[c]

Abbreviations: CNS, central nervous system; HBOC, hereditary breast and ovarian cancer syndrome; HOC, hereditary ovarian cancer; LS, Lynch syndrome; NR, not reported; PJS, Peutz-Jeghers syndrome; PPAP, polymerase proofreading associated polyposis; SCTAT, sex cord stromal tumor with annular tubules.
[a] Mutations carry an increased risk, but specific range unknown.
[b] Combined risk of renal pelvis, stomach, ovary, small bowel, ureter, and brain.
[c] Lifetime risk of any cancer 90% by age 70.

Box 2
Common hereditary cancer syndromes encountered by obstetrician gynecologists and associated clinical features: Lynch syndrome

Associated mutations
- MLH1, MSH2, MSH 6, PMS 2, EPCAM

Hallmark family history components[a]
- Multiple generations affected by Lynch-associated cancers
- Colorectal or endometrial cancer at younger ages

Associated cancers
- Endometrial cancer
- Colon cancer
- Ovarian cancer
- Pancreatic cancer
- Gastric cancer
- Small intestine cancer
- Central nervous system (particularly glioblastoma)
- Ureteral or renal pelvis cancer
- Sebaceous neoplasms

[a] Not all families meet every criteria but any of these should be explored for a possible link to Lynch syndrome.
Data from Refs.[6,14,32]

fashion. Polymerase proofreading associated polyposis is aptly named because this syndrome is most commonly associated with colonic polyps and colon cancers; however, germline mutations in *POLD1* specifically also carry an increased risk of endometrial cancer (see **Table 1**).[20–22] These cancers can mimic Lynch-associated cancers histologically and can have loss of expression of Lynch proteins on IHC and may be microsatellite unstable.

Cowden Syndrome

Cowden syndrome is caused by a germline mutation in the *PTEN* gene and is associated with an increased risk for multiple cancers (**Box 3**). Cowden syndrome is inherited in an autosomal-dominant fashion. The most common cancer associated with Cowden syndrome is breast cancer, but these patients also carry a lifetime risk of endometrial cancer of 28%.[23] Other cancers associated with PTEN mutations are thyroid cancer, most commonly the follicular thyroid subtype, and renal cancers (see **Table 1**). Cowden syndrome is also associated with hallmark physical characteristics that are helpful in the identification of these patients. These include macrocephaly (head circumference >58 cm in women), multinodular goiters, trichilemmomas, gastrointestinal hamartomas, and Lhermitte-Duclos disease.

Peutz-Jeghers Syndrome

Peutz-Jeghers syndrome, defined by a germline mutation in the *STK11(LKB1)* gene, is inherited in an autosomal-dominant fashion, and is characterized by several clinical characteristics, most notably benign hamartomatous polyps of the gastrointestinal

---

Box 3
Common hereditary cancer syndromes encountered by obstetrician gynecologists and associated clinical features: Cowden syndrome

Associated mutation
- PTEN

Diagnostic criteria[a]

Major
- Breast or endometrial cancer
- Multiple gastrointestinal hamartomas or ganglioneuromas
- Macrocephaly (head circumference >58 cm in women)
- Mucocutaneous lesions (trichilemmoma, palmerplantar keratosis, oral mucosal papillomatosis, or multiple cutaneous facial papules)

Minor
- Autism spectrum disorder or intellectual disability (IQ <75)
- Colon, renal, or thyroid cancer
- Thyroid structural lesions (adenoma, nodule, goiter)

Associated cancers
- Endometrial cancer (major criteria)
- Colon cancer (minor criteria)
- Breast cancer (major criteria)
- Thyroid cancer (typically follicular, minor criteria)
- Renal cell cancer
- Sebaceous neoplasms

[a] Patients having one major criteria and two minor merit further formal genetic evaluation for Cowden syndrome.
Data from Refs.[6,14,32]

tract, mucocutaneous pigmented macules, and increased risk of several malignancies including gastrointestinal and nongastrointestinal cancers (**Box 4**). From a gastrointestinal standpoint, colorectal cancers are the most common type of cancer, but patients remain at an increased risk of gastric cancer, pancreatic cancer, and cancers of the small bowel.[24,25] Women with Peutz-Jeghers syndrome are also at a significantly increased lifetime risk of developing breast cancer. From a gynecologic standpoint, patients are at increased risk for minimal deviation adenocarcinoma of the cervix, better known as adenoma malignum; sex cord stromal tumors with annular tubules of the ovary; and uterine cancer (see **Table 1**).[26]

Li-Fraumeni Syndrome

TP53 is known as the "guardian of the genome" and acts as an important tumor-suppressor gene by identifying cells with DNA damage (**Box 5**).[27] Thus, it is no surprise that patients with germline mutations in TP53 are at an increased risk for a multitude of cancers, most commonly bony and soft tissue sarcomas, breast cancer, adrenocortical carcinomas, and brain tumors.[28–30] Women with Li-Fraumeni syndrome are at highest risk for breast cancer and present at an early age with a median age of diagnosis of 33 (see **Table 1**).[31] There have been reported cases of uterine and ovarian cancer in Li-Fraumeni mutation carriers; however, the risk of these cancers is not nearly as high as other cancers associated with TP53 mutations.

IDENTIFICATION OF HIGH-RISK WOMEN

The first step is to evaluate women who have a prior cancer diagnosis and to evaluate every patient's family cancer history for telltale indications of a potential hereditary cancer syndrome. Hallmark signs of hereditary cancer syndromes include young age at cancer diagnosis, multiple cancers in one person, multiple generations affected, and clustering of cancer types suggestive of a particular syndrome. Particular attention should be taken to ask about cancers that correlate with known genetic syndromes, including breast, ovarian (primary peritoneal and fallopian also), endometrial, pancreatic, colon, gastric, thyroid, aggressive prostate cancer, sarcomas, and

---

Box 4
Common hereditary cancer syndromes encountered by obstetrician gynecologists and associated clinical features: Peutz-Jeghers syndrome

Associated mutation
• STK-11(LKB1)

Hallmark family history components[a]
• Gastrointestinal polyps
• Mucocutaneous pigmentation of the mouth, lips, nose, eyes, genitalia, or fingers
• Family history of Peutz-Jeghers
• Associated cancers

Associated cancers
• Gastrointestinal cancers (colon, stomach, gastric, and pancreatic)
• Breast cancer
• Ovarian sex cord stromal cancers (not epithelial ovarian cancers)
• Cervical cancer (particularly adenoma malignum subtype)
• Uterine cancer

[a] Not all families meet every criteria but any of these should be explored for a possible link to Peutz-Jeghers syndrome.
   Data from Refs.[6,14,32]

Box 5
Common hereditary cancer syndromes encountered by obstetrician gynecologists and associated clinical features: Li-Fraumeni syndrome

Associated mutation
- TP53

Hallmark family history components[a]
- Extremely young age at cancer diagnoses and multiple generations affected by associated cancers
- Classic criteria for diagnosis of Li-Fraumeni
- Individual diagnosed with a sarcoma (<45 years) AND a first-degree relative with a cancer <45 years and an additional relative with a cancer <45 years

Associated cancers
- Soft tissue sarcomas
- Osteosarcoma
- Breast cancer (especially <31 years)
- Adrenocortical carcinoma
- Leukemia
- Central nervous system cancers
- Lung cancer
- Ovarian/endometrial cancer (much less common)
- Essentially any cancer is found in these families

[a] Not all families meet every criteria but any of these should be explored for a possible link to Li-Fraumeni syndrome.
Data from Refs.[6,14,32]

melanoma. Family history should include first-degree relatives (parents, siblings, offspring), second-degree relatives (eg, grandparents, uncles/aunts, nephew/nieces, half-siblings), and potentially third-degree relatives (eg, first cousins, great grandparents). Next follows situations that might herald the need for referral to a genetic or high-risk specialist for further evaluation but if clinical suspicion is raised, referral is almost always warranted (**Fig. 1**).[6,14,32]

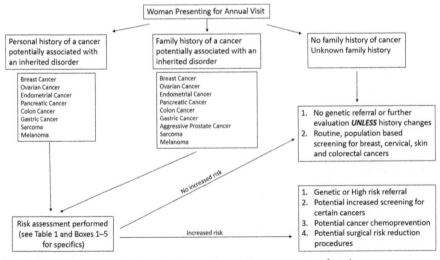

Fig. 1. Algorithm for patient evaluation and genetic assessment referral.

Women with a personal or family history of breast cancer who merit genetic/high-risk evaluation as follows:

- Potential hereditary syndromes that could be involved include hereditary breast ovarian cancer (eg, BRCA mutations and other DNA repair), Li-Fraumeni (p53 mutation), Cowden syndrome (PTEN mutation), ATM, CDH, CHEK2 mutations
- Breast cancer diagnosed younger than age 45 or diagnosed younger than 50 with another close relative with breast cancer
- Triple negative breast cancers diagnosed younger than age 60 (estrogen and progesterone and Her-2 neu receptor negative)
- Ashekenazi Jewish inheritance
- Any male breast cancer
- Family history of breast cancer in addition to any of the following: ovarian, pancreatic, aggressive prostate cancer, or multiple sarcomas

Women with a personal or family history of ovarian (or fallopian tube/primary peritoneal) cancer who merit genetic/high-risk evaluation as follows:

- Up to 24% of ovarian cancer could be hereditary and potential hereditary syndromes that could be involved include hereditary breast ovarian cancer (eg, BRCA mutations and other DNA repair) or Lynch syndrome (MSH2, MSH6, MLH1, PMS2, or EPCAM mutations)[1,33]
- Any woman with an epithelial ovarian cancer diagnosis (and most women with a first-degree relative with ovarian cancer) meets criteria for genetic testing, even in the absence of any other family cancer history
- Family history of ovarian cancer in addition to any of the following: breast, pancreatic, endometrial, colon, gastric, or aggressive prostate cancer raises suspicion further for a genetic predisposition

Women with a personal or family history of endometrial cancer who merit genetic/high-risk evaluation as follows:

- Up to 6% of endometrial cancer may be hereditary and potential hereditary syndromes that could be involved include primarily Lynch syndrome (MSH2, MSH6, MLH1, PMS2, or EPCAM mutations) but rarely Cowden (PTEN)[34]
- Women younger than 50 have a much higher rate of Lynch syndrome
- Since about 2013, many institutions are doing universal screening of all endometrial cancers for signs of Lynch syndrome (either IHC or microsatellite instability); if the cancer screens positive, the patient is referred for genetic evaluation
- Family history of endometrial cancer in addition to any of the following: colon, gastric, ovarian, breast, pancreatic, or thyroid raises suspicion further for a genetic predisposition

Women with a personal or family history of colon cancer who merit genetic/high risk evaluation as follows:

- Potential hereditary syndromes that could be involved include primarily Lynch syndrome (MSH2, MSH6, MLH1, PMS2, or EPCAM mutations) but rarely Cowden (PTEN) or others
- Since about 2013, most institutions are doing universal screening of all colon cancers for signs of Lynch syndrome (either IHC for the MMR proteins or microsatellite instability of the tumor DNA); if the cancer screens positive, the patient is referred for genetic evaluation.

- Family history of colon cancer in addition to any of the following: endometrial, ovarian, gastric, breast, pancreatic, or thyroid raises suspicion further for a genetic predisposition

Tools to evaluate/quantify genetic risk include the following:

- Breast cancer risk and risk of BRCA mutation
  - *BRCAPRO* (available at http://www4.utsouthwestern.edu/breasthealth/cagene/)
  - Tyrer-Cuzick (available at http://www.ems-trials.org/riskevaluator/)
  - BOADICEA (available at www.srl.cam.ac.uk/genepi/boadicea/boadicea_home.html)
- Increased risk of hereditary breast ovarian cancer based on family history (from NCCN guidelines) that meets criteria for genetic testing
  - Known deleterious BRCA (or other related gene) mutation in the family
  - Personal history of either ovarian or male breast cancer
  - Personal history of breast cancer and one of the following criteria:
    - Diagnosed at 45 years age or younger
    - Diagnosed at 50 years of age or younger with either an additional breast cancer, one or more close relative with breast or pancreatic, or prostate cancer
    - Diagnosed at 60 years of age or younger with triple negative breast cancer
  - Personal history of pancreatic cancer and a blood relative with ovarian or breast cancer or Ashkenazi Jewish heritage
- Risk of having a Lynch or MMR gene mutation
  - PREMM [1,2,6] model (http://premm.dfci.harvard.edu/)
  - MMRpro (available at http://www4.utsouthwestern.edu/breasthealth/cagene/ or http://bcb.dfci.harvard.edu/bayesmendel/software.php)
- Increased risk of Lynch syndrome based on family history (from NCCN Guidelines) based on one or more of the following[33]:
  - First-degree relative with colorectal or endometrial cancer diagnosed younger than 50 years of age
  - First-degree relative with colorectal or endometrial cancer and another Lynch-related cancer (gastric, ovarian, pancreas, ureter and renal pelvis, biliary tract, glioblastoma, or small intestine)
  - Two or more first- or second-degree relatives with Lynch-associated cancers listed previously and one diagnosed younger than 50 years of age
  - Three or more first- or second-degree relative at any age

SCREENING STRATEGIES

Once a patient has been identified as a mutation carrier, various screening and risk-reduction options should then be used to help mitigate cancer risk. Specific gynecologic cancer screening recommendations for each hereditary cancer syndrome are outlined in **Table 2**.

Breast Cancer Screening

Although all of the syndromes discussed significantly increase a woman's lifetime risk of gynecologic malignancies, there remains debate regarding the impact of gynecologic cancer screening on early diagnosis or cancer-related mortality. In contrast, breast cancer screening has been well defined in terms of recommendations for the high-penetrant mutations. The American Cancer Society published guidelines in 2007 for women at an increased lifetime risk of breast cancer, defined by at least a

Table 2
Recommended gynecologic surveillance and risk-reduction strategies

Gene	Genetic Syndrome	Surveillance Strategy (Age to Start)[6,14]	Risk Reduction (Age to Consider)[a,6,14]
BRCA1	HBOC	Consider Q 6 mo/annual TVUS and serum CA125 Breast awareness (18) Clinical breast examination Q 6–12 mo (25) Annual breast MRI (25–29) Annual mammogram (30)	RRSO (35–40) Discuss RR mastectomy Consider RR agent[b]
BRCA2	HBOC	Consider Q 6 mo/annual TVUS and serum CA125 Breast awareness (18) Clinical breast examination Q 6–12 mo (25) Annual breast MRI (25–29) Annual mammogram (30)	RRSO (40–45) Discuss RR mastectomy Consider RR agent[b]
BRIP1	HOC	No current recommendations	Consider RRSO (45–50)
RAD51C	HOC	No current recommendations	Consider RRSO (45–50)
RAD51D	HOC	No current recommendations	Consider RRSO (45–50)
MLH1	LS	Consider annual TVUS and/or office endometrial sampling	RRSO when childbearing complete (35–40) RR hysterectomy when childbearing complete
MSH2/ EPCAM	LS	Consider annual TVUS and/or office endometrial sampling	RRSO when childbearing complete (35–40) RR hysterectomy when childbearing complete
MSH6	LS	Consider annual TVUS and/or office endometrial sampling	RRSO when childbearing complete (35–40) RR hysterectomy when childbearing complete
PMS2	LS	Consider annual TVUS and/or office endometrial sampling	RRSO when childbearing complete (35–40) RR hysterectomy when childbearing complete
POLD1	PPAP	No current recommendations	No current recommendations
PTEN	Cowden	Consider annual TVUS and office endometrial sampling at age 30–35 Breast awareness (18) Clinical breast examination Q 6–12 mo (25) Annual breast MRI (30–35) Annual mammogram (30–35)	Discuss hysterectomy on completion of childbearing Discuss RR mastectomy
STK11	PJS	Annual pelvic examination and pap smear (18–20) Consider annual TVUS Clinical breast examination Q 6 mo (25) Annual breast MRI (25) Annual mammogram (25)	Discuss RR mastectomy

(continued on next page)

	Genetic	Surveillance Strategy	Risk Reduction
Table 2 (*continued*)			
Gene	**Syndrome**	**(Age to Start)[6,14]**	**(Age to Consider)[a,6,14]**
TP53	Li-Fraumeni	Breast awareness (18) Clinical breast examination Q 6–12 mo (20–25) Annual breast MRI (20–25) Annual mammogram (20–25)	Discuss RR mastectomy

Abbreviations: HBOC, hereditary breast and ovarian cancer syndrome; HOC, hereditary ovarian cancer; LS, Lynch syndrome; PJS, Peutz-Jeghers syndrome; PPAP, polymerase proofreading associated polyposis; RR, risk reducing; RRSO, risk-reducing salpingo-oophorectomy; TVUS, transvaginal ultrasound.
 [a] Age may be adjusted based on age of first diagnosis in family.
 [b] Tamoxifen, raloxifene, aromatase inhibitors.

20% to 25% lifetime risk by family history, or a known inherited predisposition. These guidelines incorporate annual breast MRI in addition to annual mammogram.[35] In our practice, we stagger these studies so that the patient has some form of screening every 6 months.

Ovarian Cancer Screening

No studies to date have shown a mortality impact with the addition of ovarian cancer screening in women at an increased lifetime risk of this disease.[36,37] Screening usually takes the form of transvaginal ultrasound and serum CA125 levels, despite well-documented shortcomings of both. Transvaginal ultrasound is the most sensitive imaging modality for the ovaries and is the imaging study of choice for the evaluation of a pelvic mass. Unfortunately, most pelvic masses identified in premenopausal women, the age group where ovarian cancer screening is the most useful, are benign. Identification of such masses can lead to surgical intervention with associated operative risks and loss of ovarian function.[38] Similarly, serum CA125 levels are elevated for a variety of benign conditions including endometriosis, history of breast cancer, smoking, liver pathology, or hormone-replacement therapy and are not reliable in premenopausal women.[39]

Recent studies have evaluated a longitudinal evaluation of CA125 in the individual patient using the Risk of Ovarian Cancer Algorithm (ROCA). ROCA measures the rate of change of CA125 over time rather than using a static normal cutoff value. ROCA was used in two prospective studies that were recently reported from the United States and the United Kingdom.[40,41] GOG 199, prospective cohort study, was analyzed in conjunction with a similar prospective trial by the Cancer Genetics Network. A total of 3692 women were screened with six incident cancers identified and nine occult cancers found at risk-reducing salpingo-oophorectomy (RRSO). Screening with ROCA every 3 months did show a stage shift with 50% if incident cancers diagnosed as early stage and ROCA did identify patients for further evaluation before CA125 levels reached the normal cutoff value of 35.[40] The United Kingdom Familial Ovarian Cancer Screening Study (UKFOCSS) identified 19 patients with an invasive ovarian cancer in 4000 screened women; however, six cancers were occult and only identified after RRSO. Eight of the 13 screen detected cancers still presented with advanced disease.[41]

Although the results from UKFOCSS and the combined US studies show a potential incremental improvement in screening, there is still much room for improvement. Current NCCN guidelines discuss consideration of transvaginal ultrasound and serum

CA125 levels for hereditary breast and ovarian cancer and Lynch syndrome, but do not endorse a firm recommendation for ovarian cancer screening in the high-risk population.[6] The authors of even the most recent trials that identified a stage shift emphasize that screening does not replace RRSO for these patients.[40]

Endometrial Cancer Screening

Fortunately, most endometrial cancers present with early stage disease as a result of the hallmark symptom of abnormal vaginal bleeding. However, this fact has made it difficult to identify a screening modality that could result in a stage shift or mortality impact. Screening options for endometrial cancer include pelvic ultrasound and in-office endometrial biopsy and both of these have been evaluated in the prospective setting. Patients at the highest risk for endometrial cancer include those with Lynch syndrome and Cowden syndrome. Similar to the use of ultrasound for ovarian cancer, the premenopausal patient population is where a screening test would be the most useful. Unfortunately, the endometrial stripe can vary widely because of the menstrual cycle and is not a reliable measurement in premenopausal patients. Several studies have been conducted in the Lynch syndrome population specifically and none have shown a benefit of ultrasound screening.[42–44]

The other option for endometrial cancer screening is annual endometrial biopsy. This has also been evaluated in the prospective setting and although cases of hyperplasia and cancer were identified on in-office biopsy, there was no difference in stage at diagnosis or survival when compared with patients who presented with symptoms.[42,43] Given these findings, the NCCN does not explicitly recommend this screening, but does qualify that it is an option at the physician's discretion.[14]

Cervical Cancer Screening

The human papilloma virus accounts for most cervical cancers and most women should be followed in accordance with the guidelines provided by the American Society for Colposcopy and Cervical Pathology. However, the NCCN does recommend annual pelvic examination with pap smear for women with Peutz-Jeghers syndrome.[14]

RISK-REDUCTION STRATEGIES
Hereditary Breast and Ovarian Cancer

Bilateral RRSO is the gold standard for ovarian cancer risk reduction for BRCA mutations and is recommended by age 35 to 40 years in *BRCA1* and by 40 to 45 years for *BRCA2* carriers (see **Table 2**).[6] Multiple prospective studies have demonstrated an 80% to 90% decrease in the risk of ovarian cancer and a 60% to 75% reduction in all-cause mortality for *BRCA* carriers who undergo RRSO.[45–49]

It is now thought that a large percentage of serous ovarian cancers may originate in the distal fallopian tube. Given this, there is increasing interest in salpingectomy as means of ovarian cancer prevention. A decision analysis in *BRCA* carriers showed that salpingectomy with delayed oophorectomy has a higher quality-adjusted life expectancy compared with RRSO.[50] In addition, *BRCA* mutation carriers are interested in salpingectomy with delayed oophorectomy as demonstrated by a survey reporting that up to 33% would be interested in pursuing this approach.[51] However, RRSO remains the current standard of care, and those interested in pursuing salpingectomy with delayed oophorectomy should only do so as part of one of the ongoing clinical trials (NCT02321228, NCT01608074, NCT01907789, NCT02760849). Although the NCCN does not definitively recommend risk-reducing mastectomy for *BRCA* mutation carriers, or any other hereditary cancer syndromes, they do recommend a discussion with the patient regarding the option of mastectomy.[6]

There is some evidence for an increased risk of uterine papillary serous cancer in *BRCA1* mutation carriers; however, the absolute risk is small and the role of hysterectomy for these patients remains controversial.[9] Although one benefit of hysterectomy at the time of RRSO is simplification of hormone therapy, there remains to be definitive evidence that it is useful in preventing uterine cancers.[52] Risks and benefits of hysterectomy should be discussed and the surgical decision individualized.

Use of oral contraceptives (OCP) has been shown to decrease risk of ovarian cancer specifically in women with BRCA mutations. There is obviously concern about breast cancer risk for these women, and there have been conflicting reports about correlation between OCP use and increased breast cancer risk in BRCA carriers. However, the largest meta-analysis did not identify any increased risk of breast cancer for these women.[53] The degree of ovarian cancer risk reduction is significant, with estimates with just 1 year of use ranging from 33% to 80% for *BRCA1* and 58% to 63% for *BRCA2* carriers.[54]

Hormonal therapy has also been shown to decrease the risk of breast cancer in *BRCA2* mutation carriers specifically. Chemoprevention with the selective estrogen receptor modulator tamoxifen may reduce the risk of breast cancer by 62% in *BRCA2* mutation carriers, but does not significantly decrease breast cancer risk in *BRCA1* mutation carriers.[55] This discrepancy is likely because *BRCA1* mutation carriers are more likely to be diagnosed with estrogen receptor–negative disease. Side effects of tamoxifen include vasomotor symptoms, thromboembolic events, endometrial cancer, and cataracts.[56] Raloxifene has also been studied as a chemopreventive agent in postmenopausal women with a family history of breast cancer, but not in BRCA mutation carriers specifically. In high-risk women in general, raloxifene also demonstrated a decreased risk of estrogen receptor–positive breast cancer.[57] The Study of Tamoxifen and Raloxifene (STAR) trial evaluated tamoxifen and raloxifene directly in women with a family history of breast cancer. In this patient population, tamoxifen had a greater risk reduction (relative risk of invasive cancer for raloxifene, 1.24; 95% confidence interval, 1.05–1.47); however, both agents significantly decreased the lifetime risk of breast cancer. In addition, raloxifene users had a lower risk of thromboembolic events and cataracts compared with tamoxifen users. Although not statistically significant, there were also more cases of uterine cancer diagnosed in tamoxifen users (relative risk of uterine cancer for raloxifene, 0.62; 95% confidence interval, 0.535–1.08).[58,59] A benefit/risk index was developed from the STAR trial and showed that for postmenopausal women with an intact uterus, raloxifene had a better benefit/risk index, whereas the benefit risk index was similar for both agents in women without a uterus.[60] Lastly, aromatase inhibitors have also been shown to decrease breast cancer risk in high-risk women, but not in women with BRCA mutations specifically.[61,62]

Hereditary Ovarian Cancer

RRSO for carriers of deleterious mutations in *BRIP1*, *RAD51C*, and *RAD51D* is recommended by age 45 to 50 years (see **Table 2**).[6] However, there have been no prospective studies to quantify ovarian cancer risk reduction or mortality benefit for these women. Women with these mutations are also eligible for ongoing trials evaluating salpingectomy for ovarian cancer prevention (NCT02760849). In addition, studies on the benefit of OCPs specific to these populations are lacking but their use should be considered for cancer prevention given the benefits seen in the general population.

Lynch Syndrome

Hysterectomy has been shown to decrease the risk of endometrial cancer in women with Lynch syndrome. Likewise, a benefit for RRSO at the completion of childbearing has also been supported. In a case control study of women with Lynch syndrome, there were no cases of cancer in women who underwent prophylactic surgery compared with rates of 33% and 5% for endometrial and ovarian cancer in aged-matched control subjects that did not have surgery.[63] A decision tree analysis also described an overall survival benefit for hysterectomy and RRSO in women with Lynch syndrome compared with screening or annual pelvic examination.[64] The NCCN recommends that hysterectomy with or without bilateral salpingo-oophorectomy should be considered as an option for women with Lynch syndrome at the completion of childbearing.[14] The SGO and the American College of Obstetricians and Gynecologists encourage discussion of surgical risk reduction by a woman's early to mid-40s (see **Table 2**).[65]

Salpingectomy for ovarian cancer prevention has yet to be explored for women with Lynch syndrome, although they are eligible to participate in an ongoing clinical trial (NCT02760849). There have also been no studies specifically addressing the role of chemoprophylaxis in women with Lynch syndrome. However given that in the general population there is a 50% reduction in ovarian cancer seen with 15 years of OCP use and a 24% reduction seen in endometrial cancer for every 5 years of use, OCPs should be considered for cancer prevention in women with Lynch syndrome.[66,67]

Polymerase Proofreading Associated Polyposis

There are no current guidelines for risk reduction in patients with germline mutations in POLD1; however, if a patient was identified, it would be reasonable to follow guidelines for Lynch syndrome.

Cowden Syndrome

Hysterectomy should be considered for women with Cowden syndrome who have completed childbearing (see **Table 2**).[6] Consideration of OCPs or progesterone-only methods may also be a reasonable risk-reduction strategy, although prospective data to quantify benefit are lacking. In addition, there should be a discussion of risk-reducing mastectomy with these patients including degree of risk reduction and reconstruction options.[6]

Peutz-Jeghers Syndrome

Although these women are at increased risk of ovarian, endometrial, and cervical cancers, risk-reducing surgery has not been recommended.

Li-Fraumeni Syndrome

Although patients with Li-Fraumeni syndrome are at a significantly increased lifetime risk of a wide range of cancers, including possible ovarian and uterine cancer, there are no specific recommendations for risk-reducing hysterectomy or salpingo-oophorectomy in this patient population. Patients should be evaluated on a case-by-case basis following a consideration of a detailed family history. However, given the high risk of breast cancer in the women, it is recommended to discuss the option of risk-reducing mastectomy.[6]

SUMMARY

Women with inherited risks for cancer are typically followed by their primary care physicians, including OB/GYNs, rather than cancer genetics experts. Thus, it is imperative that all physicians take enough of a cancer history to identify the warning signs of a potential hereditary syndrome and refer such individuals (and their families) to resources that could markedly improve their chances of remaining cancer free and healthy.

REFERENCES

1. Walsh T, Casadei S, Lee MK, et al. Mutations in 12 genes for inherited ovarian, fallopian tube, and peritoneal carcinoma identified by massively parallel sequencing. Proc Natl Acad Sci U S A 2011;108(44):18032–7.
2. King MC, Marks JH, Mandell JB. Breast and ovarian cancer risks due to inherited mutations in BRCA1 and BRCA2. Science 2003;302(5645):643–6.
3. Antoniou A, Pharoah PD, Narod S, et al. Average risks of breast and ovarian cancer associated with BRCA1 or BRCA2 mutations detected in case series unselected for family history: a combined analysis of 22 studies. Am J Hum Genet 2003;72(5):1117–30.
4. Ford D, Easton DF, Stratton M, et al. Genetic heterogeneity and penetrance analysis of the BRCA1 and BRCA2 genes in breast cancer families. Am J Hum Genet 1998;62(3):676–89.
5. SGO Clinical Practice Statement: Genetic testing for ovarian cancer. Available at: https://www.sgo.org/clinical-practice/guidelines/genetic-testing-for-ovarian-cancer/. Accessed October 24, 2016.
6. NCCN Guidelines Genetic/Familial High-Risk Assessment: breast and ovarian version 1.2017 2016; Available at: https://www.nccn.org/professionals/physician_gls/pdf/genetics_screening.pdf. Accessed September 1, 2017.
7. Stadler ZK, Salo-Mullen E, Patil SM, et al. Prevalence of BRCA1 and BRCA2 mutations in Ashkenazi Jewish families with breast and pancreatic cancer. Cancer 2012;118(2):493–9.
8. Mersch J, Jackson MA, Park M, et al. Cancers associated with BRCA1 and BRCA2 mutations other than breast and ovarian. Cancer 2015;121(2):269–75.
9. Shu CA, Pike MC, Jotwani AR, et al. Uterine cancer after risk-reducing salpingo-oophorectomy without hysterectomy in women with BRCA mutations. JAMA Oncol 2016;2(11):1434–40.
10. Loveday C, Turnbull C, Ramsay E, et al. Germline mutations in RAD51D confer susceptibility to ovarian cancer. Nat Genet 2011;43(9):879–82.
11. Loveday C, Turnbull C, Ruark E, et al. Germline RAD51C mutations confer susceptibility to ovarian cancer. Nat Genet 2012;44(5):475–6.
12. Ramus SJ, Song H, Dicks E, et al. Germline mutations in the BRIP1, BARD1, PALB2, and NBN genes in women with ovarian cancer. J Natl Cancer Inst 2015;107(11):djv214.
13. Tiwari AK, Roy HK, Lynch HT. Lynch syndrome in the 21st century: clinical perspectives. QJM 2016;109(3):151–8.
14. NCCN Clinical practice guidelines in oncology: genetic/familial high-risk assessment: colorectal. 2016; Available at: https://www.nccn.org/professionals/physician_gls/pdf/genetics_screening.pdf. Accessed October 11, 2016.
15. Barrow E, Hill J, Evans DG. Cancer risk in Lynch syndrome. Fam Cancer 2013; 12(2):229–40.
16. Lu KH, Dinh M, Kohlmann W, et al. Gynecologic cancer as a "sentinel cancer" for women with hereditary nonpolyposis colorectal cancer syndrome. Obstetrics Gynecol 2005;105(3):569–74.

17. Chui MH, Gilks CB, Cooper K, et al. Identifying Lynch syndrome in patients with ovarian carcinoma: the significance of tumor subtype. Adv Anat Pathol 2013; 20(6):378–86.
18. Chui MH, Ryan P, Radigan J, et al. The histomorphology of Lynch syndrome–associated ovarian carcinomas: toward a subtype-specific screening strategy. Am J Surg Pathol 2014;38(9):1173–81.
19. SGO Clinical Practice Statement: screening for Lynch syndrome in endometrial cancer. Available at: https://www.sgo.org/clinical-practice/guidelines/screening-for-lynch-syndrome-in-endometrial-cancer/. Accessed October 24, 2016.
20. Palles C, Cazier JB, Howarth KM, et al. Germline mutations affecting the proof-reading domains of pole and pold1 predispose to colorectal adenomas and carcinomas. Nat Genet 2013;45(2):136–44.
21. Briggs S, Tomlinson I. Germline and somatic polymerase ε and δ mutations define a new class of hypermutated colorectal and endometrial cancers. J Pathol 2013; 230(2):148–53.
22. Bellido F, Pineda M, Aiza G, et al. POLE and POLD1 mutations in 529 kindred with familial colorectal cancer and/or polyposis: review of reported cases and recommendations for genetic testing and surveillance. Genet Med 2016;18(4):325–32.
23. Tan MH, Mester JL, Ngeow J, et al. Lifetime cancer risks in individuals with germline PTEN mutations. Clin Cancer Res 2012;18(2):400–7.
24. van Lier MG, Wagner A, Mathus-Vliegen EM, et al. High cancer risk in Peutz-Jeghers syndrome: a systematic review and surveillance recommendations. Am J Gastroenterol 2010;105(6):1258–64.
25. Resta N, Pierannunzio D, Lenato GM, et al. Cancer risk associated with STK11/LKB1 germline mutations in Peutz-Jeghers syndrome patients: results of an Italian multicenter study. Dig Liver Dis 2013;45(7):606–11.
26. McGarrity TJ, Kulin HE, Zaino RJ. Peutz-Jeghers syndrome. Am J Gastroenterol 2000;95(3):596–604.
27. Laptenko O, Prives C. p53: master of life, death, and the epigenome. Genes Development 2017;31(10):955–6.
28. Villani A, Tabori U, Schiffman J, et al. Biochemical and imaging surveillance in germline TP53 mutation carriers with Li-Fraumeni syndrome: a prospective observational study. Lancet Oncol 2011;12(6):559–67.
29. Kratz CP, Achatz MI, Brugières L, et al. Cancer screening recommendations for individuals with Li-Fraumeni syndrome. Clin Cancer Res 2017;23(11):e38–45.
30. Villani A, Shore A, Wasserman JD, et al. Biochemical and imaging surveillance in germline TP53 mutation carriers with Li-Fraumeni syndrome: 11 year follow-up of a prospective observational study. Lancet Oncol 2016;17(9):1295–305.
31. Olivier M, Goldgar DE, Sodha N, et al. Li-Fraumeni and related syndromes. Correlation between tumor type, family structure, and TP53 genotype. Cancer Res 2003;63(20):6643–50.
32. ACOG Practice Bulletin No 182: Hereditary breast and ovarian cancer syndrome. Obstet Gynecol 2017;130(3);e110–26.
33. Norquist BM, Harrell MI, Brady MF, et al. Inherited mutations in women with ovarian carcinoma. JAMA Oncol 2016;2(4):482–90.
34. Leenen CH, van Lier MG, van Doorn HC, et al. Prospective evaluation of molecular screening for Lynch syndrome in patients with endometrial cancer ≤ 70 years. Gynecol Oncol 2012;125(2):414–20.
35. Saslow D, Boetes C, Burke W, et al. American cancer society guidelines for breast screening with MRI as an adjunct to mammography. CA Cancer J Clinicians 2007;57(2):75–89.

36. Buys SS, Partridge E, Black A, et al. Effect of screening on ovarian cancer mortality: the prostate, lung, colorectal and ovarian (PLCO) cancer screening randomized controlled trial. JAMA 2011;305(22):2295–303.
37. Partridge E, Kreimer AR, Greenlee RT, et al. Results from four rounds of ovarian cancer screening in a randomized trial. Obstetrics Gynecol 2009;113(4):775–82.
38. Fishman DA, Cohen L, Blank SV, et al. The role of ultrasound evaluation in the detection of early-stage epithelial ovarian cancer. Am J Obstetrics Gynecol 2005;192(4):1214–21.
39. Johnson CC, Kessel B, Riley TL, et al. The epidemiology of CA-125 in women without evidence of ovarian cancer in the prostate, lung, colorectal and ovarian cancer (PLCO) screening trial. Gynecol Oncol 2008;110(3):383–9.
40. Skates SJ, Greene MH, Buys SS, et al. Early detection of ovarian cancer using the risk of ovarian cancer algorithm with frequent CA125 testing in women at increased familial risk: combined results from two screening trials. Clin Cancer Res 2017;23(14):3628–37.
41. Rosenthal AN, Fraser LSM, Philpott S, et al. Evidence of stage shift in women diagnosed with ovarian cancer during phase ii of the United Kingdom familial ovarian cancer screening study. J Clin Oncol 2017;35(13):1411–20.
42. Renkonen-Sinisalo L, Bützow R, Leminen A, et al. Surveillance for endometrial cancer in the hereditary nonpolyposis colorectal cancer syndrome. Int J Cancer 2007;120(4):821–4.
43. Gerritzen LH, Hoogerbrugge N, Oei AL, et al. Improvement of endometrial biopsy over transvaginal ultrasound alone for endometrial surveillance in women with Lynch syndrome. Fam Cancer 2009;8(4):391.
44. Dove-Edwin I, Boks D, Goff S, et al. The outcome of endometrial carcinoma surveillance by ultrasound scan in women at risk of hereditary nonpolyposis colorectal carcinoma and familial colorectal carcinoma. Cancer 2002;94(6):1708–12.
45. Kauff ND, Satagopan JM, Robson ME, et al. Risk-reducing salpingo-oophorectomy in women with a BRCA1 or BRCA2 mutation. New Engl J Med 2002;346(21):1609–15.
46. Kauff ND, Domchek SM, Friebel TM, et al. Risk-reducing salpingo-oophorectomy for the prevention of BRCA1- and BRCA2-associated breast and gynecologic cancer: a multicenter, prospective study. J Clin Oncol 2008;26(8):1331–7.
47. Domchek SM, Friebel TM, Neuhausen SL, et al. Mortality after bilateral salpingo-oophorectomy in BRCA1 and BRCA2 mutation carriers: a prospective cohort study. Lancet Oncol 2006;7(3):223–9.
48. Domchek SM, Friebel TM, Singer CF, et al. Association of risk-reducing surgery in BRCA1 or BRCA2 mutation carriers with cancer risk and mortality. JAMA 2010; 304(9):967–75.
49. Finch AP, Lubinski J, Møller P, et al. Impact of oophorectomy on cancer incidence and mortality in women with a BRCA1 or BRCA2 mutation. J Clin Oncol 2014; 32(15):1547–53.
50. Kwon JS, Tinker A, Pansegrau G, et al. Prophylactic salpingectomy and delayed oophorectomy as an alternative for BRCA mutation carriers. Obstetrics Gynecol 2013;121(1):14–24.
51. Holman LL, Friedman S, Daniels MS, et al. Acceptability of prophylactic salpingectomy with delayed oophorectomy as risk-reducing surgery among BRCA mutation carriers. Gynecol Oncol 2014;133(2):283–6.
52. Hartmann LC, Lindor NM. The role of risk-reducing surgery in hereditary breast and ovarian cancer. New Engl J Med 2016;374(5):454–68.

53. Iodice S, Barile M, Rotmensz N, et al. Oral contraceptive use and breast or ovarian cancer risk in BRCA1/2 carriers: a meta-analysis. Eur J Cancer 2010; 46(12):2275–84.
54. Friebel TM, Domchek SM, Rebbeck TR. Modifiers of cancer risk in BRCA1 and BRCA2 mutation carriers: a systematic review and meta-analysis. J Natl Cancer Inst 2014;106(6):dju091.
55. King M, Wieand S, Hale K, et al. Tamoxifen and breast cancer incidence among women with inherited mutations in BRCA1 and BRCA2: national surgical adjuvant breast and bowel project (NSABP-P1) breast cancer prevention trial. JAMA 2001; 286(18):2251–6.
56. Fisher B, Costantino JP, Wickerham DL, et al. Tamoxifen for prevention of breast cancer: report of the national surgical adjuvant breast and bowel project P-1 study. J Natl Cancer Inst 1998;90(18):1371–88.
57. Nelson HD, Smith M, Griffin JC, et al. Use of medications to reduce risk for primary breast cancer: a systematic review for the U.S. preventive services task force. Ann Intern Med 2013;158(8):604–14.
58. Vogel VG, Costantino JP, Wickerham D, et al. Effects of tamoxifen vs raloxifene on the risk of developing invasive breast cancer and other disease outcomes: the NSABP study of tamoxifen and raloxifene (STAR) p-2 trial. JAMA 2006;295(23): 2727–41.
59. Vogel VG, Costantino JP, Wickerham DL, et al. Update of the national surgical adjuvant breast and bowel project study of tamoxifen and raloxifene (STAR) P-2 trial: preventing breast cancer. Cancer Prev Res (Phila) 2010;3(6):696–706.
60. Freedman AN, Yu B, Gail MH, et al. Benefit/risk assessment for breast cancer chemoprevention with raloxifene or tamoxifen for women age 50 years or older. J Clin Oncol 2011;29(17):2327–33.
61. Cuzick J, Sestak I, Forbes JF, et al. Anastrozole for prevention of breast cancer in high-risk postmenopausal women (IBIS-II): an international, double-blind, randomised placebo-controlled trial. Lancet 2014;383(9922):1041–8.
62. Goss PE, Ingle JN, Alés-Martínez JE, et al. Exemestane for breast-cancer prevention in postmenopausal women. New Engl J Med 2011;364(25):2381–91.
63. Schmeler KM, Lynch HT, Chen LM, et al. Prophylactic surgery to reduce the risk of gynecologic cancers in the Lynch syndrome. New Engl J Med 2006;354(3): 261–9.
64. Chen LM, Yang KY, Little SE, et al. Gynecologic cancer prevention in Lynch syndrome/hereditary nonpolyposis colorectal cancer families. Obstet Gynecol 2007; 110(1):18–25.
65. Committee on Practice Bulletins-Gynecology, Society of Gynecologic Oncology. ACOG Practice bulletin no. 147: Lynch syndrome. Obstetrics Gynecol 2014; 124(5):1042–54.
66. Havrilesky LJ, Gierisch JM, Moorman PG, et al. Oral contraceptive use for the primary prevention of ovarian cancer. Evid Rep Tevhnol Assess (Full Rep) 2013;212: 1–514.
67. Collaborative Group on Epidemiological Studies on Endometrial Cancer. Endometrial cancer and oral contraceptives: an individual participant meta-analysis of 27 276 women with endometrial cancer from 36 epidemiological studies. Lancet Oncol 2015;16(9):1061–70.

Moving?

Make sure your subscription moves with you!

To notify us of your new address, find your **Clinics Account Number** (located on your mailing label above your name), and contact customer service at:

Email: journalscustomerservice-usa@elsevier.com

800-654-2452 (subscribers in the U.S. & Canada)
314-447-8871 (subscribers outside of the U.S. & Canada)

Fax number: 314-447-8029

Elsevier Health Sciences Division
Subscription Customer Service
3251 Riverport Lane
Maryland Heights, MO 63043

*To ensure uninterrupted delivery of your subscription, please notify us at least 4 weeks in advance of move.

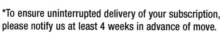
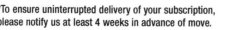

Printed and bound by CPI Group (UK) Ltd, Croydon, CR0 4YY

03/10/2024

01040391-0019